The Spirit of the Organs

The
Spirit of the
Organs

Twelve stories for practitioners and patients

John Hamwee

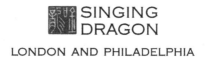

SINGING
DRAGON

LONDON AND PHILADELPHIA

First published in 2018
by Singing Dragon
an imprint of Jessica Kingsley Publishers
73 Collier Street
London N1 9BE, UK
and
400 Market Street, Suite 400
Philadelphia, PA 19106, USA

www.singingdragon.com

Library of Congress Cataloging in Publication Data
Names: Hamwee, John, author.
Title: The spirit of the organs / John Hamwee.
Description: London ; Philadelphia : Jessica Kingsley Publishers, 2017. |
    Includes bibliographical references.
Identifiers: LCCN 2017026788 (print) | LCCN 2017025677 (ebook) | ISBN
    9780857013347 (ebook) | ISBN 9781848193789 (alk. paper)
Subjects: | MESH: Medicine, Chinese Traditional | Mind-Body Relations,
    Metaphysical
Classification: LCC R601 (print) | LCC R601 (ebook) | NLM WB 55.C4 | DDC
    610.951--dc23

British Library Cataloguing in Publication Data
A CIP catalogue record for this book is available from the British Library

ISBN 978 1 84819 378 9
eISBN 978 0 85701 334 7

Printed and bound in Great Britain

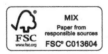

For my teachers
Meriel Darby, Angie Hicks and
Fritz Frederick Smith

Acknowledgements

Sophie Mitchell and Myra Connell have been extremely generous with the time and attention they have paid to drafts of this book and both of them have improved it hugely through their perceptive comments and suggestions. Cathy Nicholson provided much-appreciated support.

Dorsett Edmunds, Sue Newton, Viola Pemberton-Pigott, Steven Smith and Jonathan Wild all helped too.

Once again, Jessica Kingsley has been the best publisher any author could wish for.

Contents

Note to readers

The stories in this book will have particular meanings for practitioners of Chinese medicine. For readers who are not practitioners and who would like some idea of what those meanings might be, a brief description of the traditional view of the organs will help. So the Appendix contains a thumbnail sketch of the nature and functions of each organ in Chinese medicine. For the sake of brevity I have chosen to describe only those aspects of the traditional view of the organs which will illuminate the stories.

The introduction is addressed specifically to practitioners and can be safely skipped by other readers.

Introduction

Spirit

OUR PATIENTS COME TO US BECAUSE THEY know, often unconsciously, that we offer something remarkable which they sorely need. They do not want a doctor who will diagnose their illnesses as mechanical or chemical malfunctions of the body; if they did they would be content with Western medicine. Instead they want someone to see their illnesses as part of who they are, part of their lives and part of the difficulties they face in managing what is demanded of them. And although they may not have the words with which to express this kind of view, their illnesses are often disturbances of the spirit which manifest eloquently in their bodies; so in order to help them they need someone who has the theory, the concepts and the techniques to treat the body and the spirit as one.

In this materialist culture, and faced with a patient in pain or with a distressing disability, it is all too easy for acupuncturists to forget this and to start to treat the headache, the irritable bowel or the eczema symptomatically. How often, when taking a case history, does the practitioner look for disturbances not in the function of an organ but in its spirit? How often, when making an initial diagnosis, does the practitioner wonder about the state of the patient's Yi, or take time to investigate the strength of his or her Hun? And yet we know perfectly well that, as the Nei Jing puts it, 'In order to make acupuncture thorough and effective one must first cure the spirit.' Or, a more recent version of the old truth:

> ...at least in the medical tradition, Spirit is always considered to be embodied and have no independence from human life. The Chinese physician resists, both intellectually and clinically, a separation of human life into components or dichotomies; mind and body, mental and physical, soul and body, moral virtues and autonomic activities... (Kaptchuk 2000, p.66)

So to be mindful of the spirit of the organs is not some esoteric extra, of importance only to those few patients who tell you they are in existential turmoil or distress; on the contrary, an appreciation of the spirit of an organ will lead you to more accurate, more effective and more powerful treatments of the most common conditions. Indeed, as soon as you probe beneath the surface of a symptom, you quickly arrive at deep questions: Why acid reflux, for instance, when the patient's diet is exemplary and her life tranquil? Why profuse sweating only in the daytime and only on the head? Why does itching stop and start in different areas of the body at irregular intervals? And in order to answer these kind of questions the first step is to know the organs not simply as a list of functions or syndromes but as distinct aspects of the patient's spirit: one spirit with, say, twelve flavours or hues.

Traditionally, in Chinese medical thought, the spirit has five different qualities and each one is associated with an organ – Liver, Heart, Spleen, Lung and Kidney. However, in what follows I see each of these five aspects of spirit as being associated with one of the phases or elements, including both its Zang and its Fu. So, for example, I take the Yi to have aspects of both the Spleen and the Stomach, and believe that it will manifest somewhat differently depending on which of them is to the fore at any one time. Although this is not the conventional view, Ted Kaptchuk distinguishes, for example, the Yin and Yang Zhi: 'The Yang will's fear is paralyzing; the Yin will's fear is agitating and seeks to run' (Kaptchuk 2000, p.63).

The basic idea is familiar in pulse diagnosis. A practitioner may feel that the Stomach and Spleen pulses both have a slippery quality when compared with the others, and may also feel that the Spleen pulse is softer and more rounded than the Stomach. In other words, the patient's Earth energy takes on the particular quality of the Stomach and the Spleen as it moves and flows through each of them, and any difference between them will be reflected in the pulses. I think it is much the same with the spirit.

And practitioners see the Yin and Yang aspects of the spirit in everyday practice. An old man comes for treatment because he is struggling to cope with the gradual and irreversible decline in his wife's health. He may express his grief by wanting to be with her as much as possible, simply sitting quietly together for much of the day as she is hardly able to speak. Or his response may be to try to get her better; to rush about questioning her doctors, researching new drugs and arranging for some kind of complementary therapist to treat her each day. I don't think it is fanciful to see these behaviours, which I have seen in two patients, as contrasting expressions of the Po.

Some things are hard to describe: what potato tastes like, for example, or what the key of A major sounds like, or what the Yi feels like in a patient. This book tries to find a way round the difficulty by talking about the spirit of each organ not in analytical, rational, summarising language but through stories, one for each organ.

To speak of these things through stories is a very old way of describing the ineffable. If it can't be done directly then perhaps it can be done by a tale of its influence and effects. No story can be comprehensive or conclusive, and it can only be one person's interpretation of the spirit of an organ, but that doesn't matter. The point is not to try to be authoritative but to evoke your own view of that spirit and to leave you with a clearer and more practical view; one which, because you have come to it yourself, you will be able to use with confidence in the treatment room.

There's one other advantage in talking about the organs is this way – it is fun. The chapters are self-contained and can be read in any order you fancy, and you can enjoy a story and gain knowledge and insight without realising that is what is happening. For as you read you may become clear about something you have previously only half thought or half understood; or you might discover what you really think about an organ by disagreeing with its portrayal in the story. It wouldn't do as a way of learning about the functions of the organs but is the very best way of learning about their spirit – after all, the spirit never takes itself too seriously.

1

Lungs

Still life

THAT FIRST ATTACK. NEVER TO BE FORGOTTEN. Apparently some people can't breathe out. I've no idea what that's like. For me it was breathing in. It's such a peculiar feeling. Desperate signals go to the chest telling it to expand but nothing happens. It's as if a connection has been broken, the link between instinct and action. I used to have dreams of driving a car – I was only eight at the time – and I'd see some sort of obstruction ahead and slam on the brakes and there'd be that awful realisation that they weren't going to work, that the crash was inevitable and I was going to die. All in slow motion. That's when I woke up, of course, fighting for life.

It was horrible and I was very frightened, but I have to admit there was one enormous compensation. More than that actually, it was the doorway to the meaning of my life. It meant I didn't have to go to school and I could stay at home with my mother. A double bonus. I hated school and I loved being with her. And I was allowed, during the daytime, to move from my bed into hers. It was soft like her and smelled of her and from it I could see her dressing table with its silver-backed hair brush and mirror and perfume bottles and lipstick and hair pins. First things I drew actually. I think it was the reflections that fascinated me. But I'm getting ahead of the story.

So there I was, a sickly child, a mother's boy, bullied at school, who looked as if he was about to die at any minute. This was before those steroid inhalers which so many children use now. Anyway, the point is the world looks different when you might have to leave it at any minute. Hard to put into words, but everything's more intense, more itself. You look at a vase of daffodils, for instance, and you can feel the heavy bulb underground, and the fresh air above. You can't say it really, but you can paint it. Actually, I go further. Unless you have had that experience you can't really paint it.

Mother brought me crayons. I loved them in the box. The tiny gradations of colour from pale pink to deep blue. But when I used them on paper, the colours had no strength so what I drew looked feeble, as if it had been left out in the rain or bleached by the sun. It was such a disappointment, especially when what I was seeing was so vivid and alive. I kept the box on the bedside table but I stopped using the crayons. She noticed, of course. She noticed everything. And, bless her, she didn't say anything, didn't ask me to draw things for her, didn't make me feel bad for not using them, didn't even ask me what was wrong. She thought about it and she understood. And a bit later she brought me paints. Proper oil paints.

My God, those paints. Even now, after all these years, I can still feel the thrill of them. Even touching the cold metal of a tube brings it all back. And when I squeezed them what came out was thick and rich, and the colour was overwhelming and it was, praise be, a match for what I could see in my mind's eye. It was so good I didn't want to use the brushes. I thought they would thin out that fabulous gloop of colour, would smooth its impact, lose its power. That's where it came from, the technique that everyone talks about, of painting straight from the tube. People think I invented it after I broke my hand, but it's not true. It started right at the beginning.

Still lives. That's what you paint when you are bedridden, and that's what I did ever after. You can paint stillness or you can paint movement and I chose stillness. It's that pause at the end of the out breath, filled with hope, when life is about to enter once again, all over again. And in that split second before it starts, everything is pristine, untouched, clear. That's what I wanted to paint.

I gave that first picture to mother. She didn't think much of it, I know, but it's my favourite, still. Lots wrong with it, certainly, but then there's lots wrong with all the others too. But this one is the first breath, so to speak, and it shows. Somewhow I managed to get that down, the newness of it. It still shocks me, that painting. And if that's what you're after, and I am, then you can't get it back ever after, not in quite the same way, not quite as honest. Funny really. All those years, all that work, all those awards and honours and people paying enormous, ridiculous, sums of money for them, and not one of them is as good as that first one stuck in a box at the top of mother's wardrobe. A lifetime devoted to necessary failure, you might say. I might say.

You don't know which one I'm talking about? Of course you don't. You've never seen it. It's never been on show, it's not in any catalogue raisonne, it isn't reproduced in any of the books. Partly because my mother kept it in a box along with my school reports, my first teddy bear and the dreadful,

toe-curlingly smarty postcards I wrote from teenage holidays
in the rain; and partly because as soon as she died I was over
there rescuing it. Either Dad would have chucked it out with
all the rest of her stuff or brother Ian would have nicked it and
sold it, and then there would have been critics and journalists
wanting interviews and writing re-evaluations and all that
nonsense. Not that I'd begrudge him the money. I know it
must be hard for him. All his kid brother has to do is to pick
up a few tubes of paint, playthings really, and in ten minutes
bring in more money than he'll earn in a year. Or two.

Then again, that picture is unusual for being in natural
light. I did a few like that in the early days, but later I always
started work at three in the morning, so most of my paintings
have the glitter and shadows of night. The sense of being
alone, of the quiet, of the rest of the world fast asleep while
you're wide awake. All sorts of rubbish has been written
about this too, but there's a perfectly straightforward reason
for it. I used to wake at that time fighting for breath, and sleep
was out of the question. I needed a distraction, so I worked.
As soon as I pick up a tube of paint I forget everything else. It
takes so much concentration to really see what I'm trying to
get down that I don't notice my body and then, curiously, it
works better. Instinct. I love that. I wish I could paint the way a
fox runs or a kestrel hovers. Still, there's time yet to get nearer
to it. Look at Matisse in old age. Practically crippled and bedridden and what did he do? Designed the most perfect little
building and everything in it too. Did the cut outs. What a
man. I'm going to have an Indian summer like that. I've got to
start all over again anyway, now I can sleep, now I can breathe.
I can't do what I used to do, that's for sure. My pictures came
from asthma and insomnia, the both of them together, and I
don't have them any more.

It all started when I went to Turkey and got constipated. Doesn't sound much, but unless you've had it badly you have no idea how horrible it is. Not just the pain and the strain and the nasty feeling of being permanently full, replete with waste and toxic waste at that, but for the first time in my life I couldn't paint. I was like one of those whales that gets disorientated and swims up an estuary, gets beached, can't breathe, doesn't survive. I didn't know what to do with myself. How do you fill a day without work? Why would you want to?

Suddenly I was seeing the world the way everyone else sees it. Nothing remarkable at all. Chairs and tables were functional, no more. Lamplight on silver, on glass, on polished wood was convenient, distinguishing one thing from another, but that's all. Things had no beauty and gave no delight. I felt like an inmate of some mental hospital, sedated to stop him being a nuisance, gazing at the television in the residents' lounge all day long and taking in none of it.

I swallowed all the medicines I could get and they helped a bit, but not much. I was permanently bloated, waddling around like one of those white pug dogs with a sour expression on its face, my face. Always wondered why we'd picked them as a symbol of Britishness and now I knew; we are a chronically constipated race. Held in, bunged up, tight arsed.

I got quite pally with the chemist in town. He didn't speak any English and I don't speak any Turkish but we understood each other. Fellow sufferer, I think. As I came through the door, a few days after he'd given me the latest of his laxatives, he'd look up at me with raised eyebrows. I'd shake my head and he would tut in the most concerned way and plunge back into his pharmacy to find a yet stronger remedy. After we'd gone through this ritual four or five times, with increasing desperation on my side and increasing incredulity on his, he beckoned me into his office. He dialled a number, spoke to the person at the other end and then handed me the receiver. There came an English voice, calm, cultured, slightly upper class. 'I'm told you need treatment,' she said. I agreed. We made an appointment for the next day.

It was a twenty-minute drive, up into the hills behind the coast. When we got to the village the taxi driver stopped and got directions. We drew up in front of a small house on the edge of an olive grove. The front door opened and out came a woman wearing a white coat. It seemed an unlikely place for a doctor to live, let alone an English doctor, a woman in her mid-forties, I would have said, quite tall and slim, thin face, brown hair pulled back, a slight air of diffidence about her.

She took my name; obviously never heard of me. A relief in some ways. Then, after the usual questions about my medical history and the constipation, she asked me what I did for a living. I told her I was a painter (I never say artist). 'Are you working here now?' she asked. I so nearly told the conventional lie, actually one of two conventional lies. Either – 'I'm on holiday' (when I never take holidays, just go to different places to paint). Or – 'Yes, working as usual.' But for some reason I told her the truth; that for the first time in my life I'd found it impossible to put anything down on canvas.

I've thought about it a lot actually – what would have happened if I hadn't. It made me think about those completely unexpected turning points in a life when you are held suspended for a moment between two worlds, both of them possibilities. And then the moment of choice, the turn one way or the other, the fixing.

She nodded. At the time I just took it as a professional habit, a reflex action so to speak, but I know better now. Then she asked, 'Do you often wake at three o'clock?'

It's hard to convey the shock of that question. For one thing, how did she know? And for another, what possible connection could there be between my constipation and my insomnia? All that raced through my mind, but it doesn't convey the weirdness of it. To be clear, it wasn't like a medical diagnosis of bronchitis or something like that. I can quite understand that a doctor who knows what tests to carry out might find out something I don't know about one of my organs, or discover some hidden inner pathogen. That's straightforward. This was quite different.

I think my mouth must have dropped open for she said, 'I take that as a yes.' She asked a lot more questions and then told me to lie down on the couch. She picked up my right hand and touched the wrist, extremely lightly at first and then with deeper pressure, and then, after what felt like an age but was probably only thirty seconds or so, deeper still. It was an extraordinary experience. She was listening to my body, tuning in to its rhythms and flows. There was nowhere to hide. I don't care for that. I am still quite surprised I didn't get up and walk out but I suppose my intuition told me to hang on.

I sensed she was weighing up different options. Finally, she seemed to make up her mind and asked me to take off my shirt. Then she turned her back on me and busied herself at the small desk under the window. I complied. Then she bent over me and said, 'One here.' I felt nothing for a moment but then a there was a kind of tiny dull ache, a strange sensation, which was quite strong at first but faded quickly. I looked up in some astonishment. 'Oh,' she said. 'You didn't realise,

did you? I assumed the chemist told you I'm an acupuncturist.'
I didn't mind, as long as it worked.

The next morning I woke at the usual time but it was
different. Normally it's like jet lag. Ping, and I am instantly
awake, fresh and ready to start. That's why I sleep in my
clothes. Can't miss the moment. For in the first instant of
consciousness I get an idea for a picture, or sometimes its
mood, or even just a knowing of what to do with one I've
started but haven't been able to finish. It's as if my eye is
unclouded. Or perhaps it's me. In the middle of the day
I can't help wanting a picture to turn out a certain way. I
suppose I have a notion of how it ought to be. But at three in
the morning I am as a child. I play with shapes and colours,
free of inhibition or convention, the unthinking receiver of
some whispered message. The rest of the day's work is just
exploring what I've been given in that first instant.

Anyway, the morning after the treatment I woke in a
dreamlike state, feeling warm and lazy like a hibernating
animal. I took off my pullover, pulled the duvet round my
shoulders and rolled myself up into a ball. Then I drifted on
hidden currents, washed into some familiar places and off
to unknown ones, into the arms of women I've loved and
others I'd hardly met. Passive and purposeless. At one point
I found myself, brush in hand, in front of a giant canvas I
could never have painted, then standing by a Rothko which,
absurdly, I claimed as my own. But however strange each
scene or episode, the whole thing was utterly delicious, like
an unimaginable luxury. I can honestly say that I haven't felt
anything like it since I was a child in my mother's arms.

I must have fallen asleep again because the next thing I
remember was looking at my watch. It was nearly seven. The
acupuncturist had told me that I had to go to the loo at seven.

'Best time,' she'd said. 'Like swimming with the tide. Even if you don't think you need to. Might take a few days to train your body, so don't give up if it doesn't work straight away.'

As I sat on the toilet I felt desolate. Since this all began I had woken with no stimulus, no spur to make me paint. I was beginning to think it might never happen again. The despair was so acute that it was almost a physical pain. I grieved as one might mourn the loss of a guide who has led you on a long and difficult journey and who then, in the middle of the night, has silently taken down his tent, packed his belongings and stolen away. I felt abandoned in unknown country. As the full force of it hit me, I started to sob. I let out a wild animal sound, keening I think it's called. I was crying too and snotty with it. And so consumed was I by the force of all this that I hardly noticed at first; weeks and weeks of waste poured from me with no effort at all. Extraordinary.

I rang her up at lunchtime because she'd asked me to let her know how I'd got on, and anyway I wanted to thank her. I suppose I was expecting her to be ecstatic, as I was, but she simply asked me what had happened that morning. I told her. She kept wanting more detail. Was it unusual to be so hot when I woke the first time? I told her about sleeping in my clothes. Did I have the same luxurious feeling when I woke the second time as the first? Almost, not quite. Did I like Rothko's paintings? I love them. Then she said, 'Hmm...I'm not sure you're quite through it yet. If you're not right in a few days, come back. It means there's something else.'

I couldn't imagine what sort of something else there could be but I thanked her and put the phone down.

The next few days were all the same. The treatment seemed to have established a pattern. I was hugely relieved that I was better, and grateful too, but I still couldn't paint.

It was almost worse than before. I'd somehow assumed that once one thing had been put right then the rest would follow and I'd be back to normal, so when it didn't happen I started to lose heart. Would I ever work again? And if not, what kind of a life would I lead? I didn't want to be one of those people I saw on the beach and in the cafes; sixty-somethings with nothing to do for the rest of their lives but to pass the time in a meaningless routine of leisure. Might be years of it. It's not as if I was fit for anything else. I had no other talent or skill.

For the next week or so I moped around in a landscape of great beauty, wondering what to do with myself. I know it sounds ridiculous – it was ridiculous – but it took me that long to twig. This was exactly what she meant. She didn't say I might get constipated again, she just said I should go back if I wasn't right. Which I wasn't. So I went back.

This time I hired a car. I wanted to take my time and not worry about the driver fretting outside. She met me at the door as before, but her smile was a little more open and her manner less stiff.

I told her what had happened. She wrote it all down. She kept pushing me for more and more detail until I could remember no more. Then she said, 'I imagine you are still sleeping in your clothes?' I laughed out loud. It was the unexpectedness, you see. That and the sheer intelligence behind it. And I love not having to explain myself.

'Of course I am. Still hoping to leap out of bed inspired.'

Then she asked if I had a particular style. I told her about the still lives and the darkness. She wanted to know if the man in my dream was like that; she meant Rothko. I'd never made that connection before but I told her he was. Then she asked why I had stuck with one kind of painting for so long when I must be able to do anything I liked. Was it that I was averse to change, that I liked comfort and the familiar? I told her about Morandi's bottles, and how a painter can find a subject inexhaustibly interesting. 'Yes, yes,' she said, somewhat impatiently. 'But is it that you're only willing to paint in one way?'

I was struck by her question. I'd often thought that I might try something different, but whether from laziness or a frank recognition of the limits of my ability or even, as she was implying, a fear of failure, I never had. I was happy doing what I'd always done and the world approved – all of which seemed good enough at the time. But in the light of her challenge I saw the point of questioning it. Perhaps I'd given up, settled for less. I thought of Matisse and of the endlessly enquiring and adventurous spirit which lay beneath those three-piece suits, and I felt ashamed of myself.

'No. Not at all,' I replied. 'I could do something new.' I might have sounded confident but it felt like jumping off a cliff.

I got on the couch and the routine was as before but the experience was astonishingly different. The previous time I had felt nothing, or next to nothing, no more than a momentary ache each time the needles went in followed by twenty minutes or so of lying there thinking my thoughts until she announced that the session was over and I got up. This time the needles hurt more, as if I was being hit with a small blunt hammer. And then it started. The sensation was of something bubbling up – I was going to say like a fizzy drink but it was much stronger, slower and deeper than that. More like lava coming up out of a volcano. I suppose it must arise from a long way down, take some time to work its way to the surface and be, once it has started, completely unstoppable. That's what it was like, though it misses the most extraordinary and surprising bit.

For when this something or other bubbled up, it burst out onto the surface as laughter: irrepressible, uncontainable laughter. Not the sort of high-in-the-throat laughter that comes from a mental leap or surprise, nor a dry cynical laughter, but an elemental force of laughter in the depths of my abdomen, arising from some well of my being of which I was completely unaware. I tried to repress it. That worked for a moment or two, then it broke out again. Next it turned into tears, then it went back to being laughter again. It was completely beyond my control. And another thing, it wasn't my normal laugh, which is a kind of braying sound. This was more of a splutter or a giggle, the kind of noise you make when you're at some serious event like a lecture or a memorial service and you and one other person have both seen something funny which nobody else has noticed, and you keep catching each other's eye and setting each other off. That kind of laughter. Joyous, wonderful laughter, full of delight.

In the gaps, as I was trying to collect myself, I looked up to see if she was laughing too for I could hardly believe that it wasn't infectious. She wasn't, just quietly amused. I tried to apologise as well, but she brushed that aside with a shake of her head. It seemed she understood, though she offered no explanation. Eventually it died down. Then she said, 'I suggest you don't go to bed fully dressed. Not for a while anyway.'

I could see what she was getting at.

The next morning it felt very strange to wake up practically naked. Even stranger was that for the first time in years, decades, I didn't wake at three in the morning but around half past seven. The same the next day and the one after that. I was disappointed, to be honest. What was the point of sleeping through the night if there was no inspiration when I woke?

But on the fourth morning I remembered her question and my reply. Was I willing? she'd asked. I'd said I was. But if all mornings were going to be like this, and I didn't get down to work now, then presumably I never would. Dammit, I was willing. I got my paints and a small canvas. Then I thought – if it's going to be new, then let it be wholly new.

I walked to the bottom of the garden and sat down on the bench overlooking the river with the honeycombed cliffs on the far bank. It was a fine view but it didn't interest me. Then, out of the corner of my eye, I noticed an old olive tree. Its leaves were being stirred ever so slightly by a gentle breeze and that made each leaf seem distinct. It was a matter of colour, naturally, as the leaves caught the sun at slightly different angles, but there was more to it than that. It was a bit like seeing people in a crowd: all the same in one way and all individual in another. Could I paint that? Suddenly I was interested.

Half an hour later I was on my way back into town, to the chemist again. Much sign language of rubbed tummy and smiles and thumbs up persuaded him that I hadn't come for medicine; more difficult was indicating that I needed the kind of brushes women use to put on their make-up. In the end I left with five, ranging from razor thin to round and puffy. I had no idea if they would work but there was no alternative; the point was to change.

On the way back from town I saw how the breeze moved among the trees, swayed the grasses beside the road and held the birds soaring above. So I realised that when I sat down to paint my leaves I would be painting the wind – something, of course, that can't be seen. And I felt laughter stirring inside me again, that same laugh. I'd spent my life paying scrupulous attention to things, examining them in the minutest detail and then painting them, so think how ludicrous it was that I hadn't noticed the one fundamental, unalterable, essential truth – that what has to be painted is life itself. And I saw for the first time, honestly I did, that this is the point of the great still lives. They are pictures of life. I mean, how dense can you get? 'Life' is one of the two words in the title of the damn things and I hadn't even noticed.

I knew I'd never painted a great still life, of course I did, but until then I'd never known why. It's relatively easy to do apples and flowers and feathers and all that, though very far from easy, of course, but really hard to do cups and knives, linen and damask, jugs and vases. And for the first time I saw why: what has to be painted is not the thing itself but the life that went into the making of it, the life that left its unique and unrepeatable trace on the surface of the object. And I saw that I who had painted thousands of still lives, who had been feted and rewarded for doing so for the whole of my adult life, had not really painted a single one.

Can you see how funny that was? I couldn't stop smiling and every now and then I couldn't help a chuckle or two. After all, it was the best joke ever. The joke was on me, on the critics, the museums, the collectors, the connoisseurs, the dealers, the whole blooming lot of them, but most of all on me.

It took me nearly a month in Turkey to finish that little picture. I had so much to learn and I made so many mistakes as I went along, but it was one of the happiest times of my life. It was a joy to be learning again and I loved trying to work out how to paint with brushes. More than all that, the whole time was lit by that glorious joke and infused by that delicious laughter.

When it was finished I went and gave it to her. She thanked me nicely, said she liked it, was pleased I'd started to paint again, but I could tell she had no idea what she was holding in her slim hands. Just like my mother really, all over again. Not only was that little picture dynamite, at least in the art world, but it was worth a fortune too. The first of a new period and, like the only other one before, probably the best.

I never woke at three again. Nor did I ever paint another night scene. I expect you're thinking I never did another still life either, but that wouldn't be quite true. You see, I became passionate about trying to catch things in movement, a rain shower, a wave of wind across a grassy meadow, the swing of a woman's hair as she turns suddenly, a glance of love or suspicion. They were all outdoor paintings and not one was a still life, so everyone thought I was doing something new. But actually each one was life caught in a moment of stillness – and that's still life, surely? It was what I'd been after all along though no one had realised it, least of all me. You see, the joke just kept on getting better and better.

There was much theorising by the critics about the lightness of the late pictures, of the effect of using brushes and natural light, but what they were getting at was perfectly obvious if you watched people in the gallery. The pictures made them smile. I liked that. It meant that somehow or other I'd managed to paint what made me laugh all that time ago, in a small room up in the hills above the Turkish coast.

2

Large Intestine

Gold

I'LL TELL YOU WHAT I'M GOING TO DO IN MY old age, young woman, presuming I live that long, which is somewhat unlikely as a matter of fact. I'm going to be a glass blower. You think I'm too small and delicate? That I'd need hefty shoulders and a barrel chest? Well, you can't have heard me at a rally. Or, rather, you've can't have been at one of my rallies, because everyone can hear me, even above the noise of the police helicopters.

I went and got coached by an opera singer. Obviously. Those Olympic athletes, they don't expect to win unless they've put in the training. They do whatever it takes, don't they? Well, so do I. What I'm training for is far more important than a piece of cheap metal painted gold, silver or bronze.

I've never doubted the cause, you know, not once. It might not happen in my lifetime, I've always known that, but we will win. You look sceptical, young woman. You think I'm deluding myself? No, no. Right always prevails in the end.

It's a brutal world, I am well aware of that, but it's far less brutal than it was a hundred years ago. I'm looking that far ahead – of course I am. People say I'm wasting my time, banging my head against a brick wall, but they're the ones who are wasting their time fussing over food and curtains and holidays. At least I'm not doing that.

You don't want to know all this, do you? You want something personal – about early influences or how I broke away from my background or those famous lovers. Well, I'll tell you something personal, but it won't be what you expect and it might not be what you want either, but I can't help that.

Actually, now I think about it, it really started with my mother's diamond ring. I kept trying to grab it when I was a baby. I wanted to grab the rainbow in it when it caught the sun. Then later I loved that it was clear and true but it came from the depths of the earth. I loved all jewels, emeralds, rubies and sapphires, but nothing came close to diamonds. Except for glass. I do love glass.

When I was little I collected bits of coloured glass. I spent hours making patterns with them, mosaics. I never did birds or animals, just patterns. I liked turning one pattern into another so you couldn't tell how or where it changed. Ha! You didn't expect that did you? You thought I'd be all for sudden change, but you're wrong. Sudden change can flip back again, or worse. No use at all if it doesn't last.

Anyway, that first time was during a school holiday. My brothers and I had been sent to stay with my aunt and uncle in the country. They had three children too, but they were ghastly. They never talked to us, just ran wild. I don't approve. You have to learn discipline as a child or you never have it. They had a governess who pretended she was teaching them, but they hardly ever turned up. We only met at meals or when my uncle and aunt took us all out on trips – a famous temple, a zoo, a replica English garden. Terribly dull.

But one trip was not dull. My uncle had an interest in a mine and we were going to go underground with him. I thought we'd find diamonds. I was so excited I could hardly sit still as we were driven there in two enormous cars. Then we had to sit down to a meal at the mine manager's house. Went on for ever. I couldn't eat. Too excited. Even my aunt noticed. 'I do hope you're not sickening for something,' she said. 'It would be such a nuisance for the servants.' I started to explan that I was too excited to eat, but by then she'd turned away and was saying something to her hostess about the napkin linen.

The meal was over at last. We walked out onto the verandah which overlooked the entrance to the mine, quite near. My uncle and the manager walked down the steps, puffing at their cigars. I was right behind them, before all the other children.

'Rosa! Where do you think you are going?' That was my aunt. I kept going, turned over my shoulder to say, 'To the mine.'

'No, no, child. Not suitable. Come and sit down here and we women will wait for the men.'

I couldn't believe it. 'But I want to go. Please.'

'Certainly not. Now come here and if you're good we'll have a game of kaluki, won't we?' She turned to the manager's wife who immediately agreed that this was a splendid idea.

My uncle saw his wife beckoning and he saw me standing stock still and he got the whole thing wrong. 'It doesn't matter if you're not very good at Kaluki, little one,' he said. 'It'll pass the time, eh?'

There is nothing I despise more than passing the time. As if life has to be deliberately wasted.

'Off you go now,' said my uncle, 'she won't bite.'

As if that lapdog of a woman could bite anything tougher than cake. And there were the boys walking past me to the mine, taking as of right what was denied to me. They weren't even interested whereas I was desperate to go. It was so unfair and it was so wrong. Just telling you about it now, all these years later, I can still feel my fury at it. It's never left me.

My aunt and I played a couple of hands of kaluki. I couldn't be bothered to win. Then she said it had all been very tiring and perhaps she'd take a little rest. The manager's wife offered her a guest room. I said I'd be alright by myself on the verandah, so off she went. I counted to ten and then I was down the steps, across the dusty yard, and into the mine. I did wonder for a moment what was going to happen to me when they found out, but I didn't care.

The tunnel was quite wide, high enough for me to stand upright, and it was lit by a row of electric lights on a wire. There weren't any jewels. I thought the walls would be studded with them, glistening like my mother's ring, and that I would pick a few of them out for myself, but the sides of the tunnel were made of dull black rock and nothing caught the light, not even right under one of the bulbs.

After a few minutes the tunnel turned a sharp corner and dropped a few feet. I stumbled and when I looked up I found myself in an enormous cavern. It was like the mouth of a giant shark. Huge white teeth rose from the floor and loomed over me while more of them hung from the roof high above my head. In a few places the teeth met in a bite. I wanted to see what lay in the depths, but I couldn't because the bulbs were fixed to the wall at the side so I had to go round the edge.

Then the lights branched off down a side tunnel. Hanging on a peg I saw a glass lamp. I could reach high enough to take it down. Inside was a candle and matches. I lit the candle, closed the glass door and, holding it high above my head, set off into the centre of the cavern.

It was a wonderful feeling and I have never forgotten it. I was away from everyone and everything, in a place no one ever went, perhaps no one had never been, and, although I couldn't have put it into these words at the time, I loved being entirely responsible for myself.

I can't have been walking straight because at one point I looked back and couldn't see the lights any more. But I kept on because the deeper I went into the cave, the more wonderful it was. The roof got lower and lower and it was fun weaving my way between the teeth. They were different shapes too, some twisted, some bent at the top, some really thin, and a few had streaks of colour on them too, orange and gold. I touched each one as I passed and they were all different to the touch too: rough or pitted, ribbed or glassy.

And then I heard water. That was more astonishing than the teeth. Water belonged to normal life on the surface. I picked my way towards the sound. The ground went steeply down, there were no more teeth, and suddenly I was on the bank of a stream, just like an ordinary stream except, of course, it was underground. I dipped my finger in and tasted. It was water, ice-cold water, and although it was a bit different from ordinary water, it was absolutely delicious. I realised I was thirsty so I scooped it up in both my hands and drank.

The joy of it; I wish I could convey the joy of it.

I took off my shoes and socks and dipped my feet in. It wasn't deep, and although it was a bit slippery I stood up and paddled my way to the other side. It was so tempting I couldn't resist it. But I knew I should go no further. You think I am wild and reckless but as a matter of fact I always know when to stop.

I hadn't found a jewel, not a literal one, but I had found something far more precious. After that I knew that I could do what I wanted, whoever told me I couldn't, and that I'd be alright. And if one day I'm not, then it would have been well worth it for all I've done from believing I was.

That's the end of the story really. That's the something personal.

What happened next? Why, when you get to the end, do people always want to know what happened next? They want things neat and tidy, I suppose. You do? I never have.

Anyway, I found my way out alright. My uncle and the boys had long since got back. My aunt was woken to find me gone and had hysterics. They sent people off to look for me, but not down the mine, of course. So when I walked across the yard they couldn't work out how the search parties had missed me. I didn't tell them. Why should I, if they were too stupid to work it out for themselves? I just said I'd been for a walk, which was true.

But when I got undressed that night I noticed that my feet were sparkling. It was lovely. And then I saw that there were some sparkles on my hands too. I looked more carefully. I scraped at the skin and little grains came off. I collected them, put them on a piece of paper, and held them under the light. Somehow, I knew they were gold.

I didn't tell my uncle. I waited until I got home and showed my father.

'Where did you get these?'

'In the mine.'

'Did you tell your uncle?'

'No.'

'Why not?'

So then the whole truth came out. As he listened he had that look on his face which told me that he was pleased with me but didn't want to show it.

'It must have been in the water,' he said.

He gave me back my grains of gold. I thought nothing of it at the time, but now I am so grateful. He could have kept them and sold them – we could have done with the money. But it was my gold and he knew it.

So it's all there, you see. I expect you've been through all the cuttings and watched the newsreels, but I'm right, aren't I? All of it, it was all there, back then, all those years ago.

Don't look at me like that, young woman.

3

Stomach

Epiphany

SHE SAW THE HOUSE BEFORE THE VILLAGE. AS the coach came over the moor from Sedbergh she looked down the length of the valley beyond and there it was, unmistakably the vicarage. A square house with a door in the centre and two tall windows on either side, it looked as regular and orderly as a doll's house and she could imagine unclipping the front and swinging it open to reveal the rooms behind, the sitting room on one side, his study on the other. Opposite, symmetrically, would be the kitchen and dining room. Upstairs four bedrooms, one in each corner, only one of them to be occupied as yet, and the servants in the attic. The roof was a pyramid topped by two rows of six chimneys next to each other, so, she realised, the fireplaces must be in the centre of the house and not on the outside walls. It would be nice that the sitting room furniture would all face inwards. It was not as large as some of the vicarages she had known, but it was not insubstantial.

Her husband leaned over her to see out of the window
on her side of the coach. 'Will it do?' he asked, in the full
confidence that it would. For Barnaby could hardly conceive
of anywhere, or anything, that would not do. For all of his
thirty-four years he had found the world a delightful place and
the world had responded by thinking him a very good fellow
indeed. It was this disposition of his that had first attracted
Cressida to him. For she had been brought up by a chronically
anxious mother and a querulous and misanthropic father, so
Barnaby's cheerful good humour, his booming laugh and
warm heart were quite enough to win her over. She had
spent her life among clergymen and had long grown tired
of earnestness, sincerity and piety. She feared that sooner or
later she would be yoked to this combination in a husband,
but all of it was quite foreign to Barnaby's nature. As far as
she could tell, and admittedly only after a short engagement,
he regarded religion rather as other men might consider
feeding their dogs or cleaning their guns – something that
had to be done regularly and properly but which had no other
particular significance.

'It will do very well indeed,' she replied, suppressing a slight
qualm at the bleakness of the surrounding countryside and the
distance from any centre of civilisation. 'And the parishioners
are very fortunate to have someone of your Oxford education
and years of experience with the Archdeacon.'

'It's a long way from what you are used to,' he replied. 'I
do hope you will manage to settle to it.'

Cressida was touched. Not many men, in fact none of
the men she knew, would have taken the slightest interest
in what she was feeling nor had the sensitivity to realise that
this might not be entirely easy for her. 'When a woman is
taken to her own first home,' she replied, 'and by her own

new husband, she would be a most awful grouch if she were to find fault with it, particularly before she had even put a foot over the threshold.'

Barnaby took her hand and squeezed it with a gratitude which was a touch too powerfully expressed to be ideal. 'We shall do very well then, you and I,' he said. 'And you will have your piano.'

That was indeed a comfort. She might be far from the delights of Oxford and the conversation of women of accomplishment and culture, but while she had her piano she would be able to entertain and educate herself well enough.

'And you?' she asked in turn. 'You will not be preaching to scholars and churchmen any more. I fancy your sermons will have to be a good deal simpler now.' And reflecting that for the past hour she had seen nothing but small and rather mean-looking farms, she added, 'Do you suppose your congregation will be literate even?'

'Oh pooh to all that,' he replied. 'It matters not a fig that they understand a word of what I say. Church is a necessary part of their lives, like harvest or...or farrowing, er, harrowing.' She understood perfectly well that he had no idea what harrowing was. 'They come to roost, like a flock of birds, and it is simply the place to perch on a Sunday morning, or on the occasions of birth, marriage and death. In any case, most of them will take the opportunity of their one day of rest each week to fall fast asleep as I preach. Nor will I blame them for it. No, I shall address my sermons to the local landowners, and that will be no difficult matter as we shall know each other well enough from dining together. And I am quite sure that they will appreciate a brief homily each week rather than a lengthy and solemn disquisition. Apparently the previous incumbent was loquacious.'

She supposed he was right but she couldn't help being slightly shocked by his carefree attitude to what her father and his friends would have regarded as a matter of the utmost seriousness. Was it acceptable, truly, that the congregation slumbered while the ways of God were being explicated? And that their vicar would not trouble to enlighten the gentry on the doctrines of the Established Church? Still, at the same time, she could not help being aware of the advantages of such an attitude. For one thing the atmosphere in the house was likely to be more agreeable; and for another it would mean that his sermons, to which she would have to pay attention each Sunday, might be more entertaining than those to which she was accustomed. She pressed his hand, and in return he beamed at her with such an abundance of goodwill that she felt her heart respond.

The coach branched off the main turnpike and descended down a lane fringed with the glossy leaves of wild garlic. Two turns, the church towering over them on one side, the fields dropping down to the valley bottom on the other, and they drew up on a gravelled circle outside the front door. A cook, two maids, a gardener and a manservant were drawn up in a line to greet them.

There was more activity in her first two weeks at the vicarage than Cressida was accustomed to in a full year. The cook, having been used to the frugal diet of an old batchelor, was astonished at her demands, but the new wife took it as her duty to ensure that her husband was properly fed, and in any case she suspected that if she lost this battle it would be the start of a long and bitter war. Then she had to train the maids in what was expected of them and also be taken on a tour of the walled garden to discuss the produce that would be required for the vicarage. She had always taken a

keen interest in botany, and indeed would have loved to have
been a scientist like her cousin Rafe at Cambridge, so once
the gardener understood that she was genuinely interested
he told her at length what he had always wanted to do with
the garden.

Each day there were calls from the wives of local gentry
who were eagle-eyed in their assessment of her and her
housekeeping, and then there were the calls she had to make
on her social superiors, where she was judged again, though
by an entirely different set of standards. So many tests to pass
each day. And then there were the nights too. In the end, and
largely she suspected because of Barnaby's good nature, that
turned out to be less exacting than she had feared, but still
it was exhausting. She supposed it would all soon quieten
down, but in the meantime it required a certain amount
of resolution.

There was no respite until the piano had arrived and been
tuned. Then she unpacked her beloved music folios, the green
covers with their bold Teutonic lettering, and placed them one
by one in her piano stool under the tapestry seat she had so
diligently made when she was eleven years old. What would
she choose to play first, her first piece as a married woman
in her own home? She pondered the question as she leafed
through the familiar pages, genius in her hands.

With Barnaby's full agreement, she told the servants
that she was not to be interrupted from half past nine, after
she had breakfasted and given them their day's instructions,
until eleven. More eye rolling from cook and a barely stifled
grimace from Barnaby's manservant. All that changed once
she started to play. She chose the Mozart sonata she loved
most and knew best, so there were no hesitations and no
stumbles. The notes flowed from her fingers in a wild torrent

and with all of a young woman's love of life. There had been no music in that house for many a year and none of the servants had ever heard anything like this anyway. Barnaby reported that when he came out of his study he found them standing in the hall transfixed, lifted above the routine cares of their lives. After that she saw a new respect in their faces and her wishes were acknowledged with a good deal more deference than before.

And it was music that saw her through the most difficult challenge of those first weeks and months: the day the bishop came to lunch at only two days' notice. Barnaby was more anxious than she had ever seen him and she kept having to find new ways of expressing comfort and reassurance. Cook was frantic with worry about what to serve the great man. But Cressida had met bishops before and was pretty sure that he would be so used to elaborate meals which were well beyond the skill of a country kitchen that he would be glad of something simple; so she gave instructions for a hearty soup, two kinds of local cheese, home-made bread and pickles, and a pie of last year's apples from the loft.

She had to make polite conversation with his chaplain while the bishop was closeted with Barnaby in the study. When they emerged she saw to her relief that Barnaby was his normal cheery self again, although the same could not be said for the bishop. A tall thin man with a saturnine complexion and a pronounced stoop, he brought with him an air of melancholy and defeat. Cressida was shocked. He was so unlike the bishops she had met in her father's house who, without exception, appeared to relish their power and position. To this man they seemed a burden.

He greeted her courteously but his eyes were dead. Then he saw the piano.

'You play?' he asked.

This was no time for fluttering eyelashes and false feminine modesty. 'I do.'

'And which composers, may I ask?'

'Mozart, of course. Haydn, Beethoven, Schubert...'

A trace of a smile. 'Ah, Schubert. Is there a piece, I wonder...?'

'I know the Impromptus. Though it is a life's work to play them as they should be played.'

'Indeed it is.' A real smile now, and one of such sweetness that she felt a warm sympathy with the man.

'Would you, I wonder, be so kind as to play one for me? I would count it a blessing.'

'Which one would you like?'

'I would be glad if you would choose.'

She considered. A slow sad one to match his mood? Or the light ripples of joy of the F Major to lift him out of it? It didn't matter. There was sorrow and joy together in all of them; it was what she loved about Schubert.

As those first enormous chords rang out she sensed a relaxation behind her and fancied she heard a sigh. When she had finished she stood and turned round to her audience. Barnaby looked proud of her, the chaplain appeared unmoved, but tears were rolling down the bishop's face. He made no attempt to quench them, nor to mop them up with a handkerchief. He made no move from his chair, but simply sat there as the tears flowed.

The lunch was a success and afterwards she offered to play another Impromptu.

'So kind,' he said. 'So kind.'

There were more tears at the end. This time he dabbed them away and smiled at her.

'He understood, you see.' A pause. 'Thank you so much, my dear. I am very grateful.'

Barnaby escorted him out and came back into the drawing room rubbing his hands.

'Jolly good, jolly good,' he said. 'You made quite a hit there.'

'And your meeting with him? No difficulty, I trust?'

'Not a bit of it, not for me at any rate. He wanted to tell me that he has lost his faith. He thought I ought to know.'

'Poor man. No wonder.' She paused. 'And did you manage to comfort him?'

'Oh, I think so. I told him that I had never thought it was an essential in the Anglican Church. Church and State, you know. And in any case I pointed out that he would be retiring soon so it would be of no consequence then.'

Cressida was slightly shocked. 'We must invite him again,' she said.

'Good idea,' said Barnaby. 'And you could play something for him too. He seemed to like that.'

Cressida had written to her cousin at Cambridge and received back from him a formidable list of plants which he considered essential to any well-stocked English garden. She had spent happy hours looking them up in her books and then pacing the land, pondering where each should go. The kitchen garden was in good heart, lacking only an area for herbs – cook never used them – but the lawns and flower beds were sadly neglected. As the gardener observed, they lay in the shade of enormous laurels and gloomy conifers which denuded the soil and starved the straggly roses and drooping irises of much-needed light. She resolved to have them grubbed up, to open the views to south and west and to create two deep herbaceous borders which would provide welcome colour and also provide the house with cut flowers for seven or even eight months of the year.

When her plans were complete she took Barnaby for a walk though the garden one evening in late April, and pointed out how fine it would be with the improvements she had in mind. He reacted enthusiastically and made no difficulty even when she explained that the gardener would need to bring in paid hands to help with such a large job. She had been a little concerned that he might resist change on such a scale, not to mention the expense, but she ended up worrying about the exact opposite. He became enthusiastic.

It started with his idea that a small gazebo in the far corner of the lawn would be an agreeable place to sit and catch the last of the evening sun together, possibly with a glass of sherry. After that there was scarcely a day when he did not emerge from his study, red-faced and excitable, waving a plan. The least offensive was his proposal to dam the stream in the valley bottom and create a small lake: 'Jolly thing to look at and we could have a couple of hides to shoot duck'; the worst was for a formal parterre in the French style with pollarded lime trees, statues in niches and baroque fountains. The gardener said that he didn't know he could go on working there as he only knew about plants, and plants didn't seem to be what was wanted. Something had to be done.

Cressida wrote to her father saying how happy she was in her new home and how glad she was that she had married a clergyman who would be able to continue the spiritual instruction from which she had derived so much benefit in the years she had spent under her father's tutelage. However, she did have one concern and hoped that with all his years of experience he might be able to make a suggestion – as if, she thought as she dipped her pen, the old man had ever turned down a chance to tell others what to do. She was a little worried, she continued, that in so remote a district Barnaby would have no opportunity to maintain his skills in Greek and Aramaic, and there was no one of sufficient learning with whom he could discuss the pressing theological issues of the day. Such nourishment was readily available in Oxford, naturally, but not in Westmoreland.

Her father rose to the bait like a hungry trout. Have no fear, he replied, help was at hand. A colloquium planned for the following Trinity term would consider a new translation of Paul's epistles to the Romans – surely a much misunderstood man on account of the poor quality of those in current circulation – and he would beg the bishop to allow Barnaby to provide a commentary. As for theology, he liked to believe that he was quite capable of putting any man through his paces, so he was compiling a set of telling questions for Barnaby to answer which he would dispatch as soon as it was ready; having done thirty pages, he suspected that it would take only another dozen or so to complete the task.

Cressida was not an unkind woman. She also took the trouble to talk to Squire Tomlinson, the master of foxhounds, to tell him of her husband's love of hunting. 'Is that so?' he asked, looking surprised. 'The last man showed not the slightest interest, nor indeed do any of the other God botherers hereabouts.' Cressida assured him that Barnaby liked nothing more than a day following the hounds. 'Well, if he can find the time...' Cressida was sure he could find the time. 'And er...his mount...' Cressida was confident that his mount, in fact both of his mounts, were more than adequate to the task.

From then on she was free to garden as she wished. She immersed herself in books and carried on a protracted correspondence with her cousin, but she learnt most from working with the gardener. Together they improved the soil with quantities of well-rotted manure from the stables and compost from the enormous heaps in the kitchen garden which he had been building up over the years – far more than was needed for his vegetable patches, he knew, but he was not a man to let good composting material go to waste. Together they chose where to place each plant, taking full account of how much sun it would receive, how dry it would get in summer, and, it must be admitted, according to the impulse of an instinct which neither of them could quite explain but which, to their great satisfaction, they found they shared. They dug and dibbed, staked and pruned, watered and mulched and egged each other on in the way of all good partnerships.

At first the gardener had assumed that her participation was merely the passing fancy of a gentlewoman, that she was seeing the land through the rose-tinted spectacles of a town dweller come to the country, that her commitment would not survive a week of rain and mud, so leaving him to get on with things on his own as he liked and as he had always done. But after a couple of months he was happy to admit his error. Not only was she working harder, if anything, than at the start but she had a real feel for plants. She knew in a moment if one was showing signs of distress and she seemed to have an instinctive understanding of what was needed to bring it back to health. More than once, when they had disagreed on a remedy, and she had generously yielded to his knowledge and experience, it turned out that she had been right all along.

He started to seek her opinion. He had always planted his first potatoes, for example, on the second Sunday after Lent, but when he told her he was about to do so she looked a little surprised. 'You'd leave it later?' he asked. She bent down and touched the earth, then looked up at the sky and sniffed. 'I would,' she said. 'Give them a flying start.' So he held off with his potatoes and indeed it had been cold and wet for days afterwards; so when the sun finally came out and the ground became properly warm for the first time that spring, he put them in then and had his best crop ever.

It gave her a reputation in the district. As the vicar's wife, her position in society was well established and well understood, but engaging in physical work with one of the servants – when Lady Mitchinson paid a call one day, admittedly unannounced, she found Cressida with sleeves rolled up and hands caked with mud, taking turns with the gardener as they forked muck into a trench – was thought to be eccentric at best and evidence of dangerous radicalism at worst. Cressida was not sure whether to play up to it, argue her right to do what she chose in her own garden, or pretend that she was unaware of the criticism. What she was not willing to do was to stop gardening. Still, she was concerned it might cause difficulty for Barnaby so she resolved to consult him.

She chose her moment. On a balmy evening in late June they were strolling arm in arm down the newly created south walk, the scent of stocks heavy in the air and the white blooms of the newly planted roses on either side glowing more brightly than seemed possible in the dusk, when he turned to her and said, 'It is quite wonderful what you have done in so short a time. This will be a garden of great delights, a place where our children will play and vicars and vicars' wives long in the future will be able to relax after their labours, as we are doing now, and find comfort and contentment in the beauty of nature.'

It was the most poetic speech she had ever heard him make. She pressed his arm in acknowledgement and replied,

'But I fear there is a cost. Some of your parishioners, including many of those whose support for the church is essential, do not think it fitting that the vicar's wife should work herself, and alongside the gardener at that. I wonder, indeed I worry, that this might redound on you and your work.'

'Face 'em down,' was his instant reply. 'They think it worse for a lady to garden than to sit around playing cribbage and gossiping? It is better; a thousand times better.'

'Thank you.' She bowed her head in gratitude.

'When Adam delved and Eve span who was then the gentleman? Or woman? Eh?'

She smiled. 'I suspect they'd rather like it if I span.'

'Well, I'm not going to delve, so there's an end to it.' He stopped and looked around him in great satisfaction. 'However,' he went on, 'it might be wise to take more active steps. When your cousin Rafe is here in a few weeks' time you might invite Lady Mitchinson and the other harpies to tea in the garden, and ask him to conduct them on a tour of the new plants, holding forth at length about their origins and the grand houses where they were first cultivated, making sure to use all their Latin names, and generally making it clear that this is information with which a modern lady is supposed to be entirely familiar. Then, instead of harping, they'll all want to copy you.'

Cressida looked at him in frank admiration. 'That's brilliant,' she said.

'Oh, you know...'

'Just brilliant.'

'Steady on...'

He should really have been a politician, she thought. Actually almost anything but a clergyman.

Cressida put a great deal of thought into the event. The cook's homely fare would not do at all so she asked Rafe what was served at fashionable tea parties in Cambridge. Somewhat daunted, she set about collecting recipes for raspberry pavlova, plum frangipane tart, langue du chat biscuits and vanilla ice cream. The latter was especially challenging, but her aunt knew the Stricklands of Sizergh and they were kind enough to send her some ice from their ice house, well wrapped in layer upon layer of compressed straw. Then there were the teas. Farrars found her some first blush Darjeeling, as well as tippy Assam and fragrant Gunpowder from China. It would be a crime, said Mr Farrar, to make them in old teapots, stained by decades of inferior leaf, so she bit her lip and bought three new ones.

Sit the guests down first, she thought, otherwise they'd get edgy waiting for their tea and not pay attention. She'd bring them straight through from the front door, and instead of that blank wall of faded greenery, the gloomy laurels and scraggy rhododendrons, there would be light, there would be colour and there would be the fine prospect over fields and woods to the mountains of Westmoreland. She could imagine their exclamations of surprise and delight as they came through the double doors. And there would be a long table on the terrace and she would seat Lady Mitchinson right in the middle of it where she would command the view down the lawn between the two new herbaceous borders to the hills beyond.

'Will you need me to be here?' Barnaby asked, somewhat anxiously.

'Oh, I think it is a female event, don't you? Anyway, if a man is needed, I am sure Rafe will oblige.'

Barnaby looked a little doubtful at this as Rafe was not his idea of a man, but he realised it was not in his interests to raise the point. 'Just the chap,' he said.

Cressida wondered, not for the first time, how Barnaby would cope with her cousin. It was one thing to meet him in a crowd at the wedding, quite another to be his host for almost two weeks. And she could think of absolutely nothing they had in common.

The thought was made flesh when Rafe emerged from his coach, thin, stooped and pale, with wispy long hair, wearing a blue velvet cloak with a ruffled shirt beneath. Barnaby stamped up to him with a hearty smile, shook him very warmly by the hand, simultaneously clapping him on the back. Rafe reeled under the blow and his eyes flickered round as if seeking rescue. Cressida came up to him, kissed him on each cheek, and in her softest voice told him how much she was looking forward to showing him the transformation he had wrought. 'But first, you must be tired from your journey. Emily will show you to your room and then we will have tea and crumpets.'

Rafe was reassured. But not, it seemed, for long. He came downstairs almost immediately and asked if the bureau and the chaise longue in his room could be removed. Barnaby gave instructions to the staff without comment. Touched by this, Cressida gave him a smile of her warmest gratitude.

'And I have replaced the picture over the fireplace with one from the landing. Leighton.' Rafe shuddered. 'Practically pornographic.'

'Would you prefer another room?' she asked.

'Thank you, no. I've popped my nose in. They are all equally ghastly.'

Cressida had always liked Rafe so she didn't take offence. But she couldn't help glancing at Barnaby with some anxiety. He simply roared with laughter. 'It's probably all wrong for you here,' he said. 'The whole thing.'

Rafe cast his eyes to the ground and nodded.

'Is there anything in the room that is agreeable to you?' Barnaby asked.

'Frankly, no.'

Barnaby roared with laughter again. 'Tea first,' he said, 'and then we'll solve the problem.'

It turned out to be easy. Rafe loved the study. 'All those books – and no pictures, thank the Lord. The manly odour of whisky, leather and pipes. Heavenly windows. And that prospect. I shall paint it.'

So the bed was brought down to the study and Barnaby's desk was installed in the spare bedroom. From then on a curious friendship grew between the two men.

'I understand, of course, why he should be so fond of you,' Cressida commented one day to her husband, 'but I can't quite see why you are so fond of him.'

'Terrific chap,' Barnaby replied promptly. 'Tells the truth. Pretty rare, you know. And very welcome. There's too much of people being nice, far too much. So dull.'

She'd never thought of it quite like that but she knew exactly what he meant.

On the other hand, dull was exactly what was wanted with her ladies, so she approached Rafe as tactfully as she could and asked him if he would be kind enough to behave himself on the day of the great tea party. 'It means a lot to me,' she said.

His eyes widened. 'I shall play the part to perfection,' he replied.

And he did. He was by turns charming, flattering, confidential and gossipy, and he dropped names outrageously. They had never met a man like him and they couldn't get enough of it. His tour of the garden took almost two hours and not one of them complained as he talked of green carnations, explained which flowers were used in the perfumeries of Grasse and told them the secrets of the Rothschild garden at Cap Ferrat. 'Our sovereign herself,' he murmured, 'is practically an addict, you know. The hidden greenhouse at the palace. And the orangerie at Osborne. It is there she spends her happiest hours, propagating and grafting.' Instantly they all resolved to have a greenhouse and to propagate and graft themselves. 'And,' he went on, 'those with fine gardens receive the letter.'

Lady Mitchinson couldn't resist. 'What letter?'

He practically whispered, 'That she wishes to visit.'

'Because of the garden?'

'Ah...of course...you know the ways of our dear Sovereign, Lady Mitchinson. Indeed, she visits many gardens of horticultural interest. She did us the honour to grace the botanic garden which I have the privilege to serve...' Barnaby paused and looked round in a pensive way. 'And there is so much to admire here. Quite remarkable. Only the finest of sensibilities...'

A small gasp rose into the air. Mrs Tyson felt faint and the second cousin of the Earl of Lonsdale demanded a chair.

'Went well?' Barnaby asked Rafe as they sat down for dinner.

'I don't think they'll give any trouble from now on.'

'He was outrageous,' said Cressida.

That night Cressida woke early feeling hot and troubled, unable to go back to sleep. She slipped out of bed, put a coat on over her nightdress, and walked out onto the grass, relishing the cool of the morning dew on her bare feet. It was all so familiar; she had planned it all, had sown the seeds, nursed, tended and weeded every square foot, but she had never seen it at daybreak. And suddenly it felt completely different. It was when she was looking at the sweet peas clinging to a wigwam of twigs that she noticed the exact shade of violet of one flower. It was extraordinary. She had never seen colour like that before.

It was only much later that she could find words for what happened to her then, in her garden in that dawn. At the time it was simply an experience. It wasn't a thought or an idea or an emotion, it just was – like being cold or exhausted or thirsty. And, just like being cold or exhausted or thirsty, it brooked no possibility of doubt.

When she thought about it afterwards she understood what was different about her garden on that morning. Previously she had owned it. It was her creation. But now it didn't belong to her at all. The shape of each plant, its structure and energy, its leaf and bloom, the extraordinary subtlety and variety of its colouring, all of that and more, far more, was God-given. And actually not God-given, but God. In every plant, in every detail of every plant, in the old oak and the blade of grass, in the dew and the rain and the sun and the soil, in the worms and the beetles, in the sheep in the fields beyond, even in the weathered brick of the garden wall and the spade leaning against it. All that and more. Everything, in fact. And it wasn't that God was in these things, not exactly, but rather that they were different manifestations or versions of the same thing. As if God could look like this…or this…or this. In fact, like anything. Like me.

She stood astonished. Gone was her history, her personality, her place in society; gone was who she thought she was and who others took her to be, all swept away in a moment and leaving her not bereft but ecstatic. Time stopped or it went on for ever – it was the same thing.

And then came the thought – my feet are getting cold and I really should put some shoes on – and she was back, back in her normal everyday self. She looked around and everything seemed as before, not special any more. The experience was over but she wasn't the same, for she knew something she had not known before.

Had this happened to her father? Was that why he had gone into the Church? Cressida was pretty sure it hadn't happened to Barnaby, and she wondered what he would make of it – if she were to tell him, that is. For how could she explain this to someone who had not had the same experience? Imagine that he had never tasted roast lamb or listened to music – how could she possibly convey what it was like?

And what about church? Cressida had always attended dutifully, glad of the familiarity of hymns and prayers. Surely it would be different now? So the following Sunday she sat expectantly and paid particular attention to the service. But there was no hint or trace of her experience in the garden. Oddly, and somewhat aggravatingly, God appeared not to be present in his own house. Until, that is, she turned to leave at the end of the service. Then she caught the eye of Mrs Tyson in the pew behind and the woman was transformed. Normally a rather stony-faced matron with a dour expression, today light was emanating from her as if she were a lantern in a gloomy place, and she was beautiful.

I wonder what's happened to her, thought Cressida. Then she turned to greet Mrs Birkett and there it was again:

the same beauty, the same light. And then Mr Willison. Cressida thought she had better pull herself together.

She stood, a little dazed, as Barnaby came up and took her elbow. 'Alright?' he asked.

'Fine.'

Did she dare look at him?

'You look as if you've seen a ghost.'

'I have, in a way.' A slightly nervous giggle and then she glanced up at him.

Extraordinary. Even Barnaby.

So it wasn't that they'd all changed, it was her. And it wasn't that God was absent in his house, it was just that she hadn't recognised him before in each and every one of the congregation.

In the years that followed Cressida often found local society dull and restrictive, often found parishioners frustratingly narrow-minded, and sometimes longed for Barnaby to be promoted to a cathedral city where she would find companionship with women of her own education and tastes. But there was solace in her garden and satisfaction in the esteem with which she was held. For people who were in trouble or distress, who needed advice or reassurance, tended to come and see the vicar when he was out and she was in. So she was particularly busy on hunting days when it was necessary to set out chairs in the hallway for the queue. Barnaby never realised, of course, and no one ever enlightened him for fear that he would stay at home and see them himself.

Cressida never quite understood why she was so popular but she knew that it all stemmed from her experience in church. As she paid attention to petty jealousies and age-old resentments, as she saw the consequences of unthinking cruelty and careless unkindness, and as she witnessed implacable stubbornness and stupidity, she never forgot that behind it all lay the light in each one of them that she had seen that day in church, a light that was never extinguished even though, since then, it had been as invisible to her as it was to others. And so she spoke to them as no one else did, or could do, for her words were addressed to people who were not entirely stuck or trapped or despairing, people in whom lay other possibilities. Somehow, that communicated itself to them and then they could see afresh and find new hope and courage.

Some years later Barnaby was offered promotion. Many were surprised at this, but none more so than Barnaby, as he considered himself too weak in Divinity to be a Cathedral Dean. However, the new Bishop had inherited a clergy at odds with one another and a diocese riven with factions and disputes, so after deep thought, and long consultation with his predecessor, he decided that Cressida had to be brought into the Cathedral Close. As the wife of the Dean she would no doubt be able to do for the Cathedral what she had done so successfully in Barnaby's parish.

Barnaby told her about the offer, about the considerable increase in salary and the fine house they would occupy. He thought she would be glad to move to the city, to have a more cultured society and the Cathedral school nearby for their three children, so he was surprised when she seemed doubtful rather than delighted at the prospect.

She asked him if he really wanted the job.

'Well… There'll be a lot of Churchy things to do all the time. And I'll have the Bishop and the Archdeacon breathing down my neck. But it is a fine thing to be a Dean.'

'Only if you want it.'

He scratched the back of his head.

He said, 'But it's what you want, isn't it? I mean, it's the world you grew up in, the world you know…'

'I know this one now.'

'That's true.'

'And there is the garden.'

'True. I'm sure it would be a wrench. But still…'

'Don't do it for me.' She was insistent.

'Really?'

'Really. I am very happy here. Contented. We've put down roots.'

And so they stayed.

4

Spleen

Transformations

'WHAT DO YOU DO WHEN YOU ARE SEVENTY-five years old, your husband has died and your children all have busy lives of their own?' Fulvia asked her friend Lucilla as they sat over their morning coffee in the Gelateria.

'Please yourself, I suppose.'

'And when nothing pleases much any more?'

Lucilla shrugged but nevertheless gave the question serious consideration. 'Is there anything you wanted to do but never had the time, or maybe the courage? You could do that.'

Fulvia smiled, 'Talking about yourself?'

'Perhaps. But it might be true for you too.'

It was. It was Giovanni. She had not seen or heard of him for sixty years but he was still in her thoughts and prayers. 'Mushrooms and fossils,' she said out loud, without meaning to.

'Tell me.'

'Oh, I don't know. It's along time ago, and…'

'At our age everything's a long time ago.'

'That's true.' Fulvia paused. 'It was after my mother died. I was only eleven. I'd always been a sickly child but then I became asthmatic. My father didn't know what to do with me, so when I was well enough to travel, and afterwards for all the school holidays, he sent me to stay with my grandfather who lived up in the mountains. A small village, a hamlet really, near Cavello.

'Soon after I first arrived I woke one morning with a strange white light in the bedroom. At first I thought it must be snow but then I remembered that it was late in August, far too early for snow, so I got out of bed and went to the window and saw that the meadow outside had turned white overnight. I couldn't think what it was, so I went downstairs and there were lots of baskets in the hall and then grandfather came in from the kitchen and he picked up two of the baskets, small ones, and gave them to me and said, "Come on." Then he opened the old front door and led me out to the meadow and I saw that the white of the field was the white of the tops of mushrooms, thousands and thousands of mushrooms which were growing so close together that I couldn't see any grass at all between them.

'And there was Giovanni. He was already picking. I don't know what he must have thought of me. I was a fat little girl in those days, white and pasty-faced and wearing a navy linen suit, all pressed, and polished shoes. For a boy in a poor mountain hamlet, half starved just after the war, I must have looked like something from outer space.

"On your own?" grandfather asked him.

"Yes. My parents have gone to Collea for a funeral."

'Grandfather nodded. "Come to eat with us then," he said, "when we're finished."

'Backwards and forwards we went, filling basket after basket and still there were countless thousands of mushrooms on the meadow; and then other people started to arrive from nearby villages, also carrying baskets, and as the day went on and the news spread down the valley, more and more people arrived, and by the time the three of us sat down to eat there were dozens of people picking and there were still plenty of mushrooms left for everyone.

'Over the meal grandfather told us about mushrooms, how they are the fruit of an enormous underground tree and how, very rarely, when the conditions are absolutely right – it had only happened once before in all his life – all the fruit comes out at the same time, and that was what we'd been lucky enough to see. And then he showed us how to make mushroom prints. We cut off the tops and put them right way up on white paper and left them for a while; then we lifted the tops off again and there were patterns, beautiful patterns, on the paper and each kind of mushroom left a different pattern. It was like magic and we loved it.

'Giovanni came back the next day and we spent hours together drying the mushrooms very gently over the stove and then packing them carefully in bottles so they would keep through the winter for soups and stews, for the rich intense flavour, you know, and that deep colour.

'Giovanni was older than me – he must have been thirteen or fourteen – but he didn't treat me like a child. And a day or two later grandfather suggested we go out into the woods and see what mushrooms we could find for ourselves and he would tell us all about them. We came back with all sorts – tall thin white ones, red ones with white spots like in children's books, blue ones and yellow ones, frilly ones and spongy ones, ones that smelt like sweet soil and ones that stank – it was wonderful. Giovanni was so enthusiastic, so keen to bring back an abundance of mushrooms so that he could learn all about them, and I was swept up, swept along, swept away. He was the first boy I'd ever spent time with alone, or even talked to properly. He was a wonderful companion.

'Quite quickly there grew a bond between us. Perhaps it was because we were both clever. He had a very original mind, Giovanni, which swerved off and jumped about; you never knew where he'd go next. I could keep up, though. I got what he was saying and then I would add to it or amplify it or change it in some way. He liked that. And I liked dancing attendant on him, circling round him so to speak. After that, even when I was back home in Milan, he was still the centre for me and I was still in his orbit.

'You see, after mother died I was so miserable I used to hide all the time. I'd find places like inside a wardrobe in an unused room or under the fig tree with its giant leaves. But when I was with Giovanni I didn't need to hide. I felt safe. Maybe he took it upon himself to take care of me but it was more than that. He had a kind of power. You wouldn't know it to look at him, not really. He was quite short and thin, with shaggy brown hair and a quiet voice. But if you noticed his eyes, well then, then you'd know.

'As soon as I arrived at my grandfather's each summer I'd go round to see him, taking chocolate – he loved chocolate. He'd never had it before I gave him some and he couldn't get it himself, so I had to take chocolate – and he stopped whatever he was doing and we sat and talked, or walked and talked, for hours and hours.

'Then one summer he wasn't there – must have been two or three years later, so I was thirteen or fourteen. Grandfather told me he'd gone to the Ticino to stay with an aunt. It was terrible. I couldn't imagine life without him, honestly. It sounds exaggerated, I know, but I was fourteen – do you remember? The agony of that age. Grandfather said it was just a phase, that I was being a romantic adolescent, but it wasn't, and I wasn't.

'I spent the whole holiday thinking about Giovanni and about how much I missed him, and wondering whether he would be home again next holiday, and if so whether it would ever be the same again between us. Anyway, next time I went to the hamlet there he was and he seemed just the same, but that time away in the Ticino changed his life, and mine too, I suppose.

'His aunt took him to a museum one day. I've never been there but I know every single exhibit in two of the rooms; Giovanni must have told me about them a hundred times. There were displays of the geology of mountains, there were minerals and precious metals, but most of all there were fossils – and he absolutely loved the fossils. "Guess how old they are," he asked me. I decided they must be much older than I could imagine, so I said, "A million years." He laughed. "Older," he said. "Ten million," I guessed. He laughed again and I could see joy in his eyes. "Ten million is a lot, it's true. Then double it. Double it again." With each double he lifted a finger in front of his face. "Double it again. Double it again. Double it again – and that's still not enough! They are over five hundred million years old." I couldn't imagine that, but I could see how amazing it was that there were creatures on earth then and that all these millions of years later we could see what they were like.

'"And chalk," he went on, "like we use on blackboards at
school. Well, cliffs are made of it, huge cliffs. Know what it
is?" I shook my head. "Shells, that's what. Layers and layers
of the shells of sea creatures that died. It's true. And then the
Rockies in America, mountains as high as our Alps. You won't
believe it but they used to be under the sea."

'"How can they tell?" I asked.

'Giovanni gave me the most wonderful smile, I can
see it now. "No one else would have asked that," he said.
"They know because of the fossils. In the rock, two or three
thousand metres high, are the fossils of sea creatures. When
they died they dropped onto the seabed and when it was lifted
up they were lifted up too. Isn't it wonderful – to look at those
huge mountains, under snow all winter, and to know, to really
know, that they were once under the sea. That something
can change so completely that you'd never ever guess what
it used to be."

'It wasn't just about the fossils, I could tell.

'He didn't have any books and even if he could have
afforded them he wouldn't know how to go about getting
them, so I wrote to my father and a week later a parcel arrived
with two books on fossils. I expected Giovanni would flip
through them, just picking out the illustrations, but he simply
said he was grateful and then put them to one side, quietly.
"I'm going to read them properly," he said. I knew it wouldn't
be easy for him.

'The next holiday he asked me for more books on fossils,
so I wrote again. My father replied saying that apart from the
ones he'd already sent there were only technical books and
he was sure I wouldn't want them. I couldn't lie to him so I
said they were for a friend and that I would gladly forgo my
birthday present to have them. The books arrived, and this

time Giovanni blushed as I handed them to him. "I don't know what I'd do without you," he said. I told him I felt the same.

'Those books were really difficult for a boy who had only been to the village school and then only until he was ten, and there were lots of words he didn't understand. Grandfather had a dictionary and I showed him how to use it, but still there were technical terms that weren't in it, so I wrote to my father and asked him if he knew someone we could ask for help.

'A few days later my father arrived from Milan, an unheard-of event, in his big, shiny, black and white Hispano Soiuza. I felt like a spy whose cover had been blown. To a small mountain community just after the war he was alien and I wanted to belong with them and not with him.

'The whole thing was awkward. My grandfather came out of the chalet, shook his head, and greeted my father with, "What brings you here?"

'It's hard to convey the tone of his question. There was resentment and exasperation in it but affection too. I didn't know until much later that my grandfather had left Milan and the family business in disgust when it started to make uniforms for the fascists, and that my father had carried it on in spite of his express wishes. I don't think the rift was ever healed. Anyway, my father answered, "It's Fulvia. I want to know what's going on up here with this sudden interest in geology." My grandfather said, "Oh, I think she's found gold." At the time I didn't really know what he meant, but even then it pleased me.

'My father didn't come into the chalet. Looking back on it, perhaps he wasn't invited in. Anyway, he looked me up and down and said, "Introduce me to your friend." Well, Giovanni's house was tiny and poor and I couldn't imagine how his parents would cope with this visitor, so I said I'd go and fetch him. When my father saw us coming he smiled. I didn't know why he was happy about it but he was, and I was relieved to see it. He patted the bench where he was sitting, inviting Giovanni to join him, and started to ask questions: Why was he interested in geology? What fossils did he like best and why? What was he planning to be when he grew up?

'Giovanni was amazing. I admired him so much. He didn't try to impress my father or hide his lack of education. He wasn't defensive, nor was he overawed and tongue-tied. It was strange to see the two of them together – his ragged trousers and thin brown legs next to my father's immaculate light grey trousers with their knife-edged crease; my father's relaxed pose, one elbow draped over the armrest, while Giovanni sat bolt upright, the top of his head much lower than my father's shoulder.

'For a while I stood there awkwardly as they talked but then I had that familiar feeling with my father that I wasn't really wanted, so I went into the house and watched them through the window. After about twenty minutes they both stood up. My father shook Giovanni by the hand, put his head round the door and called "Goodbye", then got into his car and drove off. I went out.

'I didn't know what to say. Giovanni turned to me. "I'm going to Milan," he said.

'I couldn't believe it. "Was it my father? Did he tell you to?"

'"No, of course not. But talking to him I realised it was possible."

'"What's possible?"

'"Finding fossils."

'"What, in Milan?"

'"No, of course not. But I'll get a job there and earn enough money and then I'll go to Canada."

'"To Canada!" He might as well have said Timbuctoo.

'"Yes. They found the most amazing fossils there in a strip of shale. I told you. That was ages ago. There must be more. I'm going to find them."

'"You can't just go to Canada."

'"Yes I can. You can come too if you like."

'I shrivelled up inside. I felt like a snail which has been doused with salt. "I can't do that."

'"Why not?"

'It was one of those questions where the answer is so completely and utterly obvious that you can't think how to answer it. I stood dumbly in front of him.

'"It was my father, wasn't it?"

'He shrugged. "He asked me what I wanted to do, that was all. No one else has ever asked me that. And I knew that if I didn't leave here now and do it, I'll end up like all the others, scraping a living, knowing nothing else, learning nothing new. I might as well not have lived for all the difference it would make. Can you imagine if when…"

'"But you'd have to go to university, to study…"

'He shook his head. "You know that's not possible. But I can turn up there where they are digging, and keep on turning up until they hire me to do something, anything, whatever it is, cleaning their equipment, washing dishes, I don't care, and then I'll learn by being there and I'll do more and more and I'll end up making finds and I'll become who I want to be."

'I felt tears at the back of my eyes. Giovanni noticed and reached out both hands and took mine in his. "Stay safe," he said. "You stay safe." Then he turned away.'

Fulvia paused for a few moments then looked up at Lucillla. 'That's it really. That's the end of the story.'

'And what became of him?' asked Lucilla. 'Did he do it?'

Fulvia shook her head. 'I don't know.'

'How can you not know?'

'He left. I didn't have an address.'

'Oh, for heaven's sake, Fulvia.' Lucilla got out her phone. 'What's his name, his full name?'

'Giovanni Leone Marchetti. But what…'

'Googling him, that's what. Won't take…'

'Is that…I mean what…?'

'Really, Fulvia, there's no excuse at your age for not having a proper phone. You're perfectly capable, you just chose to ignore… Got him. Here we are. There can't be two of them. Want to see a photo too?'

Fulvia felt faint. 'Er…'

'Good-looking man still – though maybe the photo isn't all that recent. Lots of letters after his name. Looks like he made it after all – research fellow at the University of British Columbia, honorary fellow at the University of Bologna, Festschrift in his honour published by the University of Heidelberg…'

Lucilla read on from the screen in front of her but Fulvia barely heard what she was saying. Giovanni had done all that while she – she had married, had children, done a little work for the family business, had lived on one floor of the family house in Milan with her father on the floor below, and when the old man died she had moved down and her children stayed on the floor above, as if she was already half buried; while he had done all that, achieved all that, and from such a poor background without any education to speak of. She could have gone to Canada with him, could have let herself be swept up, stimulated, surprised, challenged, and instead she had chosen…what? Comfort, convenience, routine, minor pleasures – boredom. Then Lucilla said something which interrupted her train of thought.

'What, what was that you said?'

'Seems he's come home, back to Italy. You could go and see him.'

'No... No... Does it say where he lives?'

'As good as. Apparently he decided to end his days in the mountains where he grew up. You know. You could find him there.'

'Just turn up?'

'Oh, for heaven's sake, Fulvia. I thought you might be excited at the prospect. Anyone would think I was suggesting a rectal biopsy.'

'Well, I don't know. Do you think it would be alright?'

'For him or for you? He's hardly going to swoon at the sight of you and fall into your arms, saying if only he'd stayed in Milan with you all these years...'

Fulvia was annoyed. Lucilla didn't have to rub it in. Still, she couldn't help thinking that she didn't have the right to walk into someone's life like that, giving him no choice, making a claim on him simply because they had been friends sixty years before.

'Well, imagine if he did it to you,' said Lucilla, 'if he turned up at your apartment one day out of the blue.'

'It would be a shock.'

'Of course. But a nice one?'

Fulvia wasn't so sure. She wouldn't know what to say, what to do. It would be awkward, embarrassing. She could imagine his eye ranging critically around the rather over-furnished apartment, shaking his head that her life's work had simply produced these heavy unnecessary possessions, the oak chests and tapestries, the velvet curtains, the Persian rugs and French porcelain. His chalet would be bare and simple; books, of course, a few of his favourite fossils, a desk and chair.

She thought about it for six months and one spring day she went up there and knocked on his door. 'I wondered if you'd come,' he said. 'But I thought you might be dead.'

They talked for hours and then he said, 'Why not live up here? It's wonderful. The air will be good for your lungs, the views are uplifting, there are no annoying people demanding your time and attention. The villagers leave me alone except when I ask them to do something for me, when they are happy to oblige the old professor. What's so good about Milan?' She shook her head. 'Well, then. The people who own your grandfather's old chalet live in Torino and hardly ever come. They'd probably sell it to you. It'd be quite safe, you know.'

She remembered the last time he had told her to be safe. Well, she had been.

The people from Torino offered to sell the chalet at what she considered an eye-watering price, but she bought it and never regretted it for a moment. They had three years when they walked together most days and had lunch together often, but never dinner; when they collected mushrooms each autumn and invited the villagers in for a feast; when they read the same books and discussed them, often heatedly, for their tastes were very different. Then she died suddenly of a massive embolism and was buried, as she wished, in the woods behind her chalet. He is still alive and still challenging the conventional wisdom of the fossil record.

5

Heart

Mr Spencer

WHEN THOMAS SPENCER WAS A BOY HE HAD a long walk to school each day and his shoes always let in the rain, so he was prone to colds in the head and phlegm in the lungs. His father wasn't sure if schooling was worth the bother and would have rather the lad stayed home and helped him with his coal round, but his mother insisted so that was that. Thomas wasn't sure which side of the argument to take. On the one hand he hated the walk and he wasn't in the least bit interested in most of the lessons; but on the other hand he was fascinated by numbers. In his very first year he could do complicated addition and subtraction in his head, and in his second he was working out sequences of primes and asking his teacher to explain the patterns they made. Maths had never been Mrs Mitchell's strong point and she realised she couldn't keep up with him, so she got him books on square roots, then trigonometry and finally calculus. He found them easy.

When Thomas was thirteen the headmaster called him into his study and said that Dewhirsts were looking for a bright boy to start in the cashier's office and he had told them that young Spencer was very good with figures. It was an opportunity, no doubt about that. As Thomas well knew, it was the biggest firm in the area and if he worked hard it was a job for life. It would be too far to walk from home each day, so he'd have to live in digs in the week. Thomas didn't know what digs were but not having to walk to work would be wonderful.

That night he told his parents and asked them what to do. They explained about digs, told him they would miss him, but said that it was a wonderful thing for him and that it would be a step up in life. 'You'll not need to get yourself dirty with coal all day,' said his father, 'and if you keep your nose clean you'll have a lot better than what we've ever had.' Thomas looked round the familiar kitchen and wondered what better would be.

After two weeks at Dewhirsts he was bored with the job. All he had to do was copy the amounts of invoices into one book, ticking them off when they had been settled, and copy bills into another with the date they were paid. At the end of the week he had to total it all up and give the books to the chief cashier. He was allowed a whole afternoon to do it and it took him less than fifteen minutes. When he handed over the books at the end of the third week he asked if he could go home. Arthur Smedhurst, the chief cashier, took out his watch and looked at it with excessive astonishment. 'At two thirty, young Tom? What you thinking of? You go home at five and well you know it.'

So, to keep himself occupied, Thomas decided to go though the account books and calculate the difference between income and expenditure each day, each week and each month. It still wasn't five o'clock so he got our previous books and did the same for the past five years too.

As he walked home for the weekend, in the rain again, he mulled over what he had noticed. There were patterns in the figures, certainly, and he was pretty sure that there were more than he had noticed so far. What was more, he thought that the patterns told a story, one which he could deduce simply from what was in those books. He didn't have to go down onto the factory floor, nor watch goods being moved in and out of the warehouse, and he suspected that he didn't even have to know about the chief cashier's arrangements with the bank. There was much more to do, more to investigate, but he realised that the patterns would tell him things which perhaps no one else knew.

By the end of a fortnight he had worked out that there were seasonal peaks and troughs in the business. Sometimes, and with predictable frequency, there was cash to spare, while, equally predictably, some bills were paid when there was little or none, needing an overdraft from the bank. He produced a graph which showed the fluctuations and, cutting across them, a straight line which represented the business being run with no debt and no credit. One more week and he had worked out how to manage things so that it ran pretty much along that straight line. He showed his graph and conclusions to the chief cashier.

Arthur Smedley had started at Dewhirsts as the youngest clerk, just like Thomas, and had worked his way up to chief cashier. It was the height of his ambition and the height of his competence. Untrained in any mathematics, he was shrewd enough to recognise Tom's natural gift for the subject, so he took the graph home and looked it over. He was impressed. At the next opportunity he showed it to the Chairman, Isaac

Jowett Dewhirst himself, who was impressed too. Arthur Smedley was a fair man and he said it was entirely Tom's work.

Mr Dewhirst called Thomas into his office.

'Sit down, young man.' The chair was too big for him. Sitting right on the edge, he looked even younger than his thirteen years and the Chairman found it hard to believe that it could be all this lad's own work. But when he had received completely satisfactory answers to all the objections he could raise, there could be no doubt. Mentally deciding to make better use of Thomas than as a junior clerk in the cashier's office, he said, 'Credit where credit's due; you'll not find us slow in acknowledging what you've done for the business. But back to work now.' Then a thought struck him. 'Unless there is anything else you have to say.'

That's when Thomas gave him his idea for reorganising the warehouse.

A year later he had his own office and he set about solving his greatest problem – the hated walk to and from home each weekend. It was not along a main road so there were no carriages, and a horse was out of the question. The only possible answer was one of the new contraptions which he had read about in the newspaper, so he sent off for one. It wasn't clear to him why it would be much of an improvement on walking, but according to the reports it was both faster and easier. Sitting on a seat slung between two wheels, the perambulist's feet touched the ground on either side, allowing a normal walking gait, and then, apparently, the wheels amplified the natural power of the legs. As long, he discovered, as the perambulist didn't fall off.

But after a few days he was pretty skilled at it and he was delighted to discover that it cut his journey time by more than half. He got used to people laughing at him and small boys running alongside, asking to have a go. It was a success but Thomas thought there was plenty of room for improvement.

A year or so later he heard about a Frenchman who had added a mechanism by which the legs drove the front wheel of the machine. He called it a velocipede. It sounded right, it sounded faster, and Thomas wanted one. He asked everyone he encountered if they knew someone who spoke French and that led him to the door of Agnes Sorrell, the schoolteacher. She wrote a letter for him to Monsieur Michaux in Paris.

He had to wait a long time but the velocipede finally arrived at Dewhirsts and the whole office turned out to watch him ride it. They were disappointed. Getting on it was the first problem as the front wheel was over five feet high and the saddle was perched on top of it. Two strong men from the warehouse lifted him up, and were immediately thrown to the ground as the contraption fell onto them. Thomas was thrown over their heads and landed on the cobbled yard. He did it three times. Mr Dewhirst was watching from an upper window and sent a message that he wanted to see Thomas in his office immediately.

'What did you pay for that blasted thing?'

'Ten pounds, sir.'

'Ten pounds! I must be paying you too much. Anyway, you've wasted your money. I forbid you to try to ride it.'

'But, sir…'

'I need you in one piece, young man. Your notions have boosted the profits of this business by not far off twenty per cent in the past year. That's why you can afford to buy that contraption. So I'm not having you killing yourself on it – off it, more like.'

Thomas went back to Agnes and she wrote another letter to Monsieur Michaux asking for instructions. Over the

Whitsun week, when the business was closed, Thomas took the velocipede, a stepladder and the instructions which Agnes had translated, out to a cornfield which had a path running through it. On the Monday morning, having paid compensation to the farmer for the loss of his crop for about three yards on either side of the path, and having rubbed witchhazel on his bruises, in fact over virtually the whole of his body, he took it out on the road and covered ten miles in not much more than an hour. It was fantastic and he was triumphant. People gawped as he passed. Word got back to Mr Dewhirst and on the Tuesday morning he summoned Thomas into his office.

'Is it true you can ride that machine?'

'Yes, sir.'

'I ordered you not to.'

'Yes, sir.'

'Ever ignore my instructions at work?'

'No, sir.'

'Hmmm. Think there's money to be made from these things?'

'No, sir. They're too hard to ride.'

'Alright.'

That was the problem. Thomas pondered it long and hard. In the end he realised it all came down to one thing: the pedals should turn the back wheel not the front. It was as simple as that. Then everything followed. The front wheel would not have to be so big, and the saddle could be low enough so the feet could touch the ground when the machine was at rest, making it easy to mount and dismount; also, if the rider did fall off, he wouldn't hurt himself. Then the front wheel could be reserved for steering, which would put the handlebars in the right place for comfort. The saddle could be between the wheels, aiding balance and allowing a more efficient transmission of force to the pedals. Then too... but the list was endless. It was blindingly obvious – once he had thought of it – and it was right. The only trouble was that he couldn't see how to get it to work. But one day, he knew without a shadow of a doubt, his idea would become standard all over the world. One day no one would ever think that a velocipede could work in any other way.

He never forgot his problem and it was always in the back of his mind. That's when he met Hans Renold.

Mr Dewhirst had asked Thomas to go to Manchester to look through the books of a small engineering business in which he had an interest. Hans Renold, a Swiss engineer, had recently taken it over and it was Thomas's job to make sure that it was financially sound and honestly run. In his later years, reminiscing about his life and times, Thomas always used to say that Hans Renold was the most impressive man he had ever met, and that was no small tribute considering the household names with whom he became familiar.

After almost two days in the cramped and noisy office above the factory floor, Thomas completed the last of his checks, closed the account books and yawned. He could get the last train back to Skipton if he got going. He turned to Herr Renold. 'I am delighted to say that all is in order and I can give the business a clean bill of health.'

'Clean...?' Herr Renold's English did not extend to colloquial expression. Thomas explained.

'Ah. Already I know this.'

'Yes, I'm sure. But I had to reassure Mr Dewhirst, you see. Anyway, job done, so I'll be on my way.'

'But the factory. You must look, no?'

'No. I don't think so, thank you. I've been through the accounts. It's all here.' He patted the books.

Herr Renold shook his head.

'But the people. The work. The machines. This is where to see health or illness.'

'Well, I suppose…'

'Come.' There was urgency in Herr Renold's voice. 'Come. Learn.'

And learn Thomas certainly did.

Over the next few years Herr Renold taught him about the importance of well-made ball bearings, about fork rake and the wrapover stay, but he never showed him anything more crucial than the bush roller chain. He had invented it in order to drive machinery for the cotton mills and it had never occurred to him that it might have other uses. But that evening Thomas saw instantly that it was the solution to his problem – or rather the fundamental problem which had dogged the development of the velocipede from the very start. With one of Herr Renold's chains it became possible to drive the rear wheel as he had envisaged. Every velocipede – no, every bicycle – would have such a chain. Every bicycle in the whole wide world.

Thomas spent a sleepless night and the next day he went to see Mr Dewhirst. Having confirmed that all was satisfactory in the engineering works, he went on and told him of the enormous importance of Herr Renold's invention. 'If you remember, sir, I told you there was no money to be made out of the machine I ride. Well, there is incalculable money to be made from a similar but redesigned machine, using Hans Renold's bush chain to drive it.'

Mr Dewhirst had often worried that Thomas was becoming obsessed with his machine, and this seemed to confirm his fears. Profit, yes. A healthy profit, certainly. But not, not ever, incalculable. That was sheer fantasy. He wondered if the young man needed a holiday.

'Did you tell Herr Renold all this?'

'No, sir. I felt it right to tell you first.'

Mr Dewhirst thought for a minute. After all, he did have twenty per cent of Herr Renold's business and he couldn't overlook something which might increase its value. 'Very well. You have my permission to tell him.'

When Thomas showed Herr Renold his drawings of a rear-wheel-driven bicycle the engineer immediately suggested a host of improvements. It was a dazzling display of inventive genius. Every one of the ideas he thought up on the spot later became standard on practically every bicycle in the world. 'You should make bicycles yourself,' Thomas said. 'They will be everywhere. Everyone will have one.'

Hans laughed. 'Who is the best maker of bicycles?'

Thomas mentioned James Starley and Alfred Reynolds.

'Good. I will tell them. They will make better machines. I will sell more chains. I know my work; they know theirs.'

Thomas often pondered these words. But for their wisdom he might have left Dewhirsts and started a business himself making bicycles. Certainly cycling had boomed and largely due to him, though only Hans knew how instrumental he had been. But he understood that he was neither an engineer nor an entrepreneur, and that he was at his best when bringing out the best in others.

These were good years for Thomas. He succeeded Arthur Smedley as chief cashier, he learnt German in order to help Hans in his business, he married Agnes and he organised and subsidised one, then two, then three of the new omnibuses to take children to and from school.

One day, when Thomas was in his early forties, Mr Dewhirst called him into his office and told him that he had been unwell for some time and had decided to retire early in order to enjoy whatever time was left to him.

'If I could have my way, I'd hand over to you. Heaven knows you've made us a lot of money and there's plenty more to come. But it's a family business, Tom, as well you know, so I have to give it to my son who can no more run a company than I can ride one of your infernal machines. Blithering idiot. I'm not going to ask you to work for him and I can't give you any shares either, so I'll tell you what I am going to do.'

Mr Dewhirst paused to light a cigar. 'Against doctor's orders but never mind that.'

He looked up at Thomas. 'I seem to remember that you take a similar attitude to orders – when they are stupid, that is. Always liked that about you.'

Thomas suddenly realised how much he was going to miss his old boss. Not once since the day he stood in this very room, shivering with fear that he was going to be sacked for riding his velocipede, had Mr Dewhirst ever let on that he had thought well of Tom's disobedience.

'A few years ago I lent five hundred pounds to a young man, Simon Marks by name. You'll not remember; it was a personal loan, didn't go through the books. That's because it was a bad bet, on paper. But there was something about that young man, just like there was something about you, that made me want to back him. And I was right. He paid me back with interest, on the nail, two years to the day later. I've kept an eye on him ever since and unless I am very much mistaken he's going to have a bigger business than this one day.' Mr Dewhirst nodded as if agreeing with his own perspicacity. 'Last week he came to me for another loan, five thousand pounds this time. Good bit bigger, eh? Wants to expand. Quite right. He's learnt his trade and he's ready to grow to the next level. I refused.'

Mr Dewhirst paused and with deliberate care knocked the ash off his cigar into the bronze tray on his desk. He's enjoying this, thought Thomas. Spinning it out for sheer pleasure, like an actor slowing down his words when he knows he has the audience enraptured.

'I told him that I would give him the money for a fifty per cent share. No loan. What do you think of that, eh?'

'If you think it's a good arrangement, sir, then I am sure it is.'

'Oh, it's a good arrangement alright. And he accepted. He also accepted my one condition.'

Mr Dewhirst tried to wait but his enthusiasm burst out.

'That he take you as equal partner. That fifty per cent, it's yours. I'm giving it you. Credit where credit's due – I said that to you once before, didn't I? And by the way, his warehouse won't cope with the expansion. Nor will his office. You'll have to reorganise it all. But you can do that, and let him get on with the selling. Bloody good retailer he is.' It was the first time Thomas had ever heard Mr Dewhirst use a swear word. 'And I think the two of you will get along famously; him out front and you in the back. Pantomime horse. Simon Marks and Thomas Spencer.'

6

Small Intestine

Lady Mary

LADY MARY WORTLEY MONTAGU WAS A remarkable woman. Born towards the end of the seventeenth century into the very pinnacle of the English aristocracy, she broke every rule, took every risk and always told the truth – even to herself.

'Without being a jot wiser than my neighbours I have the particular misfortune to know and condemn all the wrong things I do.'

This one sentence gives a flavour of her sharp and ironic wit. On a visit to York where she encountered the local marriage market, as she called it, she commented, 'Love being as much forced up here as melons.' And as for her elevated status in the world, 'I hate the noise and hurry inseparable from great estates and titles, and look upon them as blessings that ought only to be given to fools, for 'tis only to them that they are blessings.'

So it is not altogether surprising that as a young woman she did something which was completely unacceptable in her society, and started a correspondence with a man. In her first letter to him she wrote with astonishing frankness.

> Perhaps you will be surprised at this letter. I have had many debates with myself before I could resolve on it. I know it is not acting in form but I do not look on you as I do on the rest of the world, and by what I do for you, you are not to judge my manner of acting with others... My protestations of friendship are not like other people's. I never speak but what I mean...

Meanwhile, her father, as was perfectly normal and proper at that time for a daughter of her status, had chosen her future husband – the somewhat unfortunately named Clotworthy Skeffington. Lady Mary simply refused to marry him. Her father was enraged. He insisted, she defied him. He threatened, she pleaded; she offered to promise never to marry, she was willing to be cut off financially – no small matter when it would have meant a life of relative poverty. Her friends were unsympathetic, telling her she was not being prudent. She responded, 'Prudent people are very happy; 'tis an exceeding fine thing that's certain, but I was born without it and shall retain to the day of death the humour of saying what I think.'

At the same time her father found out about her correspondence with another man. Incandescent with rage at her behaviour, he made her promise not to write any more and practically locked her up until her wedding day with Clotworthy Skeffington. She foiled him by escaping, then eloping with and marrying the man to whom she had been writing, Edward Wortley Montagu. They remained married for the rest of their lives, a relationship of great mutual affection and respect.

When her husband was appointed ambassador to the Ottoman Empire she said she was going to go with him to Constantinople, overland and in winter, and with a small child in her arms. No one believed she would actually do it, but she did, and enjoyed it all hugely. Here is a story from that time – when reading it, remember that this is the daughter of a Duke and the wife of an Ambassador.

> ...and asking him to show me his apartment I was surprised to see him point to a tall cypress tree in the garden, on the top of which was a bed for himself, and a little lower one for his wife and two children, who slept there every night. I was so much diverted with the fancy I resolved to examine his nest nearer, but after going up fifty steps I found I still had fifty to go, and then I must climb from branch to branch with some hazard of my neck, I thought it the best way to come down again.

She may have bottled out, but imagine the faces of her entourage as they watched her disappear upwards, craning their necks and worrying about how they were going to tell the Ambassador and the Sultan if she fell off.

All this is by way of introduction to a woman who might be considered a slightly more than usually wilful and eccentric aristocrat. But there was much more to her than that. She had a fierce intelligence which she trusted completely and she took one vital decision which almost all of her contemporaries thought was utterly mad, and she was proved right. Indeed, she was so far ahead of her time that what she chose to do became legally compulsory in England many years later.

The story starts with the death of her brother when he was only twenty years old, leaving a wife and two very young children. He died of smallpox. The disease begins with a high fever and then the spots come out – though calling them spots is deeply misleading. They look like nothing so much as a hive of bees or a colony of ants, temporarily stilled, and they cover the face entirely so the sufferer becomes literally unrecognisable. They itch appallingly and weep pus. The membranes of the mouth and throat, nose and eyes, swell up and make both breathing and seeing difficult. Then comes delirium, pain throughout the body and death.

She was not alone in witnessing this devastation for it was a common experience at the time. There were regular smallpox epidemics and huge numbers of people contracted the disease – everyone would have had family or close friends who had succumbed. Some people survived, about two-thirds of those infected, though, tragically, the proportion was very much lower for small children. Even those who recovered were affected for life. When the spots departed they left deep scars on the face, the pock marks, which must have been especially upsetting for young women, whose fortune, as they used to say, depended on their looks. Possibly worse were the eye problems which plagued most of the survivors, some of whom were blinded.

So when, at the age of twenty-six, Lady Mary contracted the disease herself she knew what was in store for her. She survived the ordeal, though her face, which many reported as very beautiful indeed, was badly scarred. She suffered from inflammation of her eyes for the rest of her life and she lost her eyelashes for ever.

For the next part of the story the scene shifts to Constantinople. During her time there she took delight in studying the culture and customs of Ottoman civilisation. She learned the language, wore Turkish clothes, visited Turkish women in their homes and took particular interest in the position of women in that society. Unlike most travellers from the West, she made no assumptions about the superiority of European life, and set about finding out the truth. She was surprised and impressed to find that, unlike in England where the wife's dowry, like all her property, was vested in her husband, married women in Turkey retained full ownership and control of their assets. In this spirit of open-minded enquiry she visited the baths and delighted in the fact that the women, including those of high rank, all went naked. Still, even at her hostess's urging, she could not be persuaded to go naked herself. There was a limit even for her.

All this led her to take seriously one of their more unusual customs. She found out that in September every year the women gave a party for their children.

...when they are met the old woman comes with a nutshell full of the matter of the best smallpox and asks which vein you please to have opened. She immediately rips open that which you offer her with a large needle (which gives no more pain than a common scratch) and puts into the vein as much venom as can lie on the head of her needle and after binds up the little wound with a hollow bit of shell... The children or young patients play together all the rest of the day and are in perfect health until the eighth. Then the fever begins to seize them and they keep to their beds two days, very seldom three. They have very rarely above twenty or thirty in their faces, which never mark, and in eight days time they are as well as before their illness...

In other words, she had come across what we now call
inoculation. Before continuing with the story, it is worth
pausing to consider why, although this practice had long been
common in Turkey and other countries, it had not been taken
up in Europe where smallpox was so devastating a disease.

First of all, for example, the Chaplain to the Embassy
was of the unshakeable opinion that it was an unchristian
operation and would therefore only work with infidels.
Although this seems absurd to us now, the prejudice against
Muslims was very strong, and indeed persists in some ways
in the West almost three hundred years later. Also, it must
have been hard to accept that what untrained women did was
right when it contradicted the opinions of the best doctors
of Europe – a potent combination of both sexist and racist
prejudice. And finally, given her own experience of the
virulence of the disease, it must have taken some courage
to consider, as she did, putting the venom into her son
deliberately, and to be persuaded that what was so toxic could
in fact be benign.

But courageous she was and persuaded she was, so she had
her son inoculated. It is hard to imagine the reactions of her
family and aristocratic contemporaries when they discovered
what she had done, but I expect it confirmed everything they
had ever thought of her. There is no record of her husband's
opinion – he was away at the time – but my instinct is that
he trusted her. She held off inoculating her daughter as she
realised that the child would be infectious for a short time
and her nurse had not had the disease, but it was done some
years later.

When she came back to England she kept quiet about
it for a while, but in 1721, when the next epidemic swept

the country, she could remain silent no longer. For among her own society it killed first Lady Hester Feilding, her sixteen-year-old cousin, then the Duke of Rutland, then two of his daughters, then Lady Louisa Berkley and Lord Irwin. And thousands more, unknown to her as to us.

I imagine her considering how to make the most impact. She would start at the top, naturally, and what bigger splash than the inoculation of the heir to the throne, the future king? And his mother, Princess Caroline, was not only a friend but a highly intelligent woman interested in the latest scientific advances of the day. She agreed to have it done to her children. In modern terms you'd call it a public relations coup.

She followed that up with a powerful article in the *Flying Post,* which not only set out the Turkish evidence for inoculation but also waged war even on those doctors in the West who were willing to inoculate. That was because they insisted on seeing it as a supplement to their existing, and ineffective, treatments of purgatives, fasting and bleeding. In a very modern-sounding passage she told the doctors that:

> their long preparations only serve to destroy the strength of the body, necessary to throw off the infection. The miserable gashes that they give people in the arms may endanger the loss of them...and the cordials that they pour down their throats may increase the fever to such a degree as may put an end to their lives...'tis in the power of a surgeon to make an ulcer with the help of a lancet and plaister and of a doctor to kill by prescriptions.

As a result she was savaged in print, shunned by those who would once have curried favour, and insulted in the street. Referring to 'some sanguine traveller from Turkey', which can only be Lady Mary, a leading doctor could hardly believe that 'an experiment practised only by a few ignorant women, amongst an illiterate and unthinking people, should on a sudden...so far obtain in one of the politest nations in the world as to be received in the Royal palace'.

She persisted in spite of it all and would not have been surprised to know that less than a hundred years after her death the inoculation of children against smallpox was made compulsory in England, though she might have wondered why it took them so long. Still, I doubt she could ever have thought the day would come, as it did in 1979, when the World Health Organization announced that, thanks to inoculation, smallpox had been completely eradicated.

Her life was never dull but it was electrified when, at the age of forty-seven, she met Francisco Algarotti, a man young enough to be her son. He was handsome, charming, clever, a scholar, scientist and wit. At that time he was engaged in an adaptation into Italian of Sir Isaac Newton's great book *Optics*. Soon after he arrived in London he was elected a Fellow both of the Royal Society and of the Society of Antiquaries, and he later joined the court of Frederick the Great of Prussia, champion of enlightenment thinkers, who was so impressed with him and his work that he made Algarotti a Count. Plenty of men had fallen head over heels in love with Lady Mary, including Alexander Pope, the leading poet of his age, and she had certainly loved before, but she had never fallen like she fell for Algarotti. As ever, she told herself the truth.

My reason makes me see all its absurdity, and my heart makes me feel all its importance. Feeble reason! which battles with my passion and does not destroy it, and which vainly makes me see the folly of loving to the degree that I love without hope of return.

So she had no illusions when she set about leaving England for Venice in order to be with him. When she arrived he didn't join her there, and it was almost two years later that they met in Turin. They probably never lived together, and when they parted there was no contact between them for some years. Still, her passion never abated and their later correspondence had the flavour of an old and deep friendship.

So, for the sake of what seems to have been a fleeting relationship, she left her life in England, her friends and family, and only returned many years later when she knew she was dying. Was it worth it? Did she ever regret not growing old with her husband? Through the whole of her life she made choices which seemed irrational or even crazy at the time, choices which broke the conventions of her class and era, and which had profound consequences for her and others. Were they good choices?

Questions like these may miss the essence of the matter. What people think they want may be quite different from what they actually want – let alone need. And the gifts of a period of unhappiness or struggle in our lives, so hard to perceive at the time, may become apparent many years later. How to distinguish between what is good for us and what is not?

And then there is the whole business of the head and the heart. I suppose most people would see her utter conviction of the benefits of inoculation against smallpox as the product of a sharp and lucid intelligence. But remember that she had fallen in love with Turkey, with its clothes and customs, its attitudes and values.

> ...these people are not so unpolished as we represent them. 'Tis true their magnificence is of a different taste

from ours, and perhaps of a better. I am almost of the opinion that they have the right notion of life, while they consume it in music, gardens, wine and delicate eating while we torment our brains with some scheme of politics; or studying some science to which we can never attain...

And most of all she fell in love with its women. She admired their beauty and refinement, their warmth and companionship, and was a little envious perhaps of their status and position in society.

...he and all his brethren writers lament on the miserable confinement of the Turkish ladies who are (perhaps) freer than any ladies in the universe... They go abroad when and where they please. 'Tis true they have no places but the bagnios, and there can only be seen by their own sex; however that is a diversion they take great pleasure in.

So it may not be far-fetched to see her initial enthusiasm for a practice carried out by women and among women as, at least initially, a matter of the heart.

And then there is her extraordinary passion for a man twenty-three years younger than herself and who was never going to stay with her and share her life. This was clearly a matter of heart rather than head. But does that mean she was wrong to do it, that it was a mistake in some sense, and that she would have been better, happier, to relapse gracefully into the luxurious life of an upper-class grandmother of her time? Keats (1817) wrote, 'I am certain of nothing but the holiness of the heart's affections...' Perhaps that enormous outburst of love for Algarotti can best be seen in this way: as a kind of spiritual journey which, like all such journeys, involves the abandonment of all that is comfortable and familiar, the dismay of family and friends, and the start of a new kind of life.

Perhaps she was simply foolish. Or perhaps, as with her passion for inoculation, she had the most remarkable power of discernment.

7

Bladder

The line

PARCEL 42 WAS THE ONLY ONE TALL ENOUGH to lean over the parapet so it was he who climbed the church tower to take the group photograph. It was Ninette, of course, who had the idea of putting them not in the usual serried ranks but in a line, in the original line, and the only way to get them all in the picture was from on high – hence the tower. There was some confusion as only a few of them knew their place, and there were dreadful gaps where people had been captured, but finally Ninette called out to Parcel 42 that they were ready, At the last moment, through some collective instinct, they all reached out and clasped hands. Forever after, that was the famous image of the line.

There were fifty-three of them in the photo. Most of them knew none of the others and only a few of them knew more than one or two, often by voice alone, but they were bound together by an unbreakable bond. For they had shared the most intense experiences imaginable and they knew, as no one else could possibly know, what it was like to live in constant fear. Even the parcels who had been passed down the line, and who had certainly experienced fear themselves, had no idea how the fifty-three had endured it.

The parcels may have had lectures on escape and evasion, but nothing could have prepared them for the reality. One minute they were Allied airmen only an hour or two from RAF Tangmere, bacon and eggs in the mess and a pint in the pub with the WAAFs, while the next they had parachuted down onto foreign soil, in the dark, often injured, surrounded by the enemy, knowing no one, not speaking the language and at least seven hundred miles from the border with Spain – the only feasible route home. Without help from the fifty-three, they would not have escaped capture.

Although most of them who had come to this reunion wore medals, and some wore many, they knew they were not the heroes. It was the men and women in the line who were the heroes. Day after day, year after year, they had gone hungry, given away their clothes, spent endless nights on cold benches, trains or mountain passes and faced the imminent possibility, or more accurately probability, of incarceration and torture, risking their lives and those of their families in order to help complete strangers. For as they sheltered the young men who had been shot down over enemy territory, and as they passed them like parcels down the long line of helpers through occupied Belgium and France, they lived with the constant fear of the arrival of the Gestapo, men who took mothers from their babies, who visited appalling cruelty on even the families of anyone suspected of helping the enemy and who, when they knew perfectly well that the war was over, burned a French village and all its inhabitants in it.

★ ★ ★

Henri took his place at the top of the line. He was only seventeen when he glanced out of his bedroom window one dark night and thought that there seemed to be something wrong with the sycamore tree at the end of the meadow. He went to investigate and there he found a man dangling twenty feet from the ground, the ropes of his parachute caught in the branches. Henri went back to the house, got a knife, climbed into the tree and cut the ropes. He put the man in his own bed and slept under the kitchen table.

In the morning his father kicked him awake, asking, 'What are you doing here?' Henri explained. 'Stupid boy,' his father shouted. 'Do you want to get us all killed? Get him out of the house this minute and never ever do that again.'

'No.'

His father made for the door but Henri was too quick and barred his way.

'If he goes, I go.'

'Go then. And let the Nazis deal with you if that's what you want.'

Henri took the man to his grandmother's home thirty miles away. 'But of course,' she said, and from then on there was rarely a time when her house did not shelter an Allied airman while arrangements were being made. Each of them would need clothes, forged identity papers, train tickets, money and the instructions which would lead him to the next contact along the line. It all took time to organise, and it had to be done with immense care for there were informers everywhere. And there were nosy neighbours who noticed if you bought an extra loaf from the boulangerie or when you went down to the garden shed once too often. Some of them were enthusiastic collaborators, though most did it to get a bit more food or a travel pass, or to try to save a son from being sent to Germany as slave labour.

Henri was young – some people thought too young for the responsibility – but he had a remarkable ability to see trouble; the bridge that appeared to be undefended but wasn't, the flash of greed in the eye of a sympathiser offering help, the ticket collector with an unusually military bearing. He even saw, somehow, that the two men who arrived at his grandmother's door, wearing genuine R.A.F. uniform, speaking English and asking for help, limping as though from a rough landing, were in fact Gestapo. Without a moment's hesitation he shook his head and closed the door on them. If he had not, if he had even given them a drink, he would have been taken and the line would have collapsed right at the start.

Henri looked at the people snaking away from him and saw Françoise just beyond Jacques. So that was who had taken Parcel 42 through Paris. He'd often wondered.

* * *

The first thing Françoise had noticed about him was that he was very good-looking – and still was, she thought, as she waited for him to take the photograph. She liked tall men and those with a somewhat grave air. But he was stiff upper lip, as she supposed Englishmen always were, and she smiled as she remembered their meeting at the Gare de Lyon. She had waited, hidden behind a pillar, until the concourse was busy and his back was turned, and then ran towards him, catching him by the elbow and lifting her face to be kissed. His expression was priceless. She dug her fingers into his arm by way of warning and said, 'Ah, cheri. Enfin.' He collected himself quickly, smiled and bent down to kiss her on the cheek. She turned her head so that their lips met. Then she tucked her arm under his and, chatting away with all her news, she walked him past the soldiers who always stood at the station entrance, on the lookout for men on the run.

Had she been frightened, she wondered? Certainly there were plenty of times later when she had been, when her legs were weak under her and it took all the strength she could muster to keep a tremble out of her voice. But that first time? She thought not. In those early days before her natural vivaciousness had been drained away through lack of food, of sleep, of hope, and before anyone had been arrested, she had felt invulnerable. An illusion. But she'd survived the worst they could do to her, the prison at Fresnes, Ravensbruck concentration camp. Looking up at him now, she wondered if he knew.

★ ★ ★

As they stood there, waiting for the photograph, Marcel turned to Jean Paul.

'I never met him, of course, never met any of them, but I remember him alright. Almost enough material for two men. I thought, how am I going to make him look inconspicuous, all two metres of him? Then I had an idea – go the other way. Make him stand out more. Like a Count or a Baron. So I did a pin-striped suit, double breasted, in the finest cloth I could get my hands on. Work of art it was. Must have worked alright because here he is. I'll ask him later – still got it, sir? I'd love a photo.'

'I remember that suit,' said Jean Paul. 'Thank God they got the information back to me. They didn't always, you know.

I might have made him a Flemish miner or a Dutch train driver. Can you imagine? They'd have taken one look at the papers I'd forged, then at him, and they'd have arrested him on the spot. So I made him the Director of the Rijksmuseum. Not bad, eh? Didn't speak German, naturally. Been sent South to choose which of the pictures from Provence should be stolen by the Boche and shipped back to Berlin – the Matisses and Picassos and Renoirs. Van Gogh, naturally. I did first-class tickets for the train. Never done it before. I enjoyed that. The thought of him reclining in comfort while the soldiers who were hunting him were on wooden benches in third class. Ha!'

'That suit was nearly the death of me,' said Marcel. 'I used to take the clothes I'd made round to the back room of the laundry and leave them there. That way I'd never meet whoever took them to the parcels. I'd just got to the door with the suit over my arm when they swooped. Sheer bad luck. Whistles blew and the place was swarming with soldiers. They closed off the street at both ends and threw everyone who happened to be there in a truck and took us off for questioning. I didn't think they were looking for me, for anyone in particular; it seemed like a random round-up, hoping to find something. But I wasn't sure. And how was I going to explain the suit I was carrying?

'Me – "I was doing alterations for a client."

'Boche – "Oh really? And who is it in Evingny-sur-Marne who is two metres tall and wears a pin-striped suit?"

'I went cold with fear. For Zizette more than for me. If they worked out what I was doing, they'd arrest her. And she knew, of course she knew. What they'd do to her – it terrified me. At first I panicked, like a rabbit running backwards and forwards across the road until it gets run over, but by the time they got to me I was ready. I wasn't taking the suit; I was collecting it. So simple, once I'd thought of it. It had been cleaned there before the war, had never been claimed, and no one knew who it belonged to. Maybe he was dead. So they'd given it to me to make into clothes for the children. I didn't think they'd bother to follow it up, but if they did, I was sure the people at the cleaners would have the sense to back me up. That was my worst moment actually.'

* * *

Agnes had been lucky. A few days before she was going to take three parcels on the train down to the South, she went to the Gare D'Austerlitz to get a ticket to visit an elderly aunt in Rambouillet. At the guichet they questioned her closely. Did she not know there was a new regulation in force from that day, that she needed a different permit to travel? She said she rarely took the train, told them about her aunt, convinced them that it was a simple oversight. They told her to apply at the Kommandant's Office in town. She turned to hurry away. She had to get a new travel permit urgently and take it to Claude so he could forge copies in time for the parcels who would be arriving soon.

As she turned away, she saw a very tall man on the platform opposite. She knew immediately that he was a parcel – she'd seen enough of them to know the signs – in fact, he was one of a group of three queuing to show their tickets at the barrier manned by German soldiers. She watched in horror. They wouldn't have, couldn't have, the new permits. They wouldn't survive a minute's questioning. Fear swept down her body in a wave, leaving her paralysed. She had never felt fear like this. It was as if she was feeling the fear of them all, of every single person who had helped the parcels, all the escorts and the owners of safe houses all along the line, and those like Claude in the background, all the people who were constantly waiting for the moment that was about to happen here, the moment when it all collapsed and they were left naked and helpless.

As they reached the barrier, a man stepped in front of them, papers in hand. He must be the courier. Agnes didn't know him, but that was normal; it was safer that way. He looked right – relaxed, normal – while the parcels behind him shuffled their feet and gazed vacantly around, as instructed. He was good, no doubt about that, but how would he act when they arrested him? There was nothing he could he do, but perhaps, just possibly, he might somehow be able to talk his way out of it. Then. She simply couldn't believe it. The German soldiers gave his papers a cursory glance and waved him through, waved them all through.

But they didn't have the new permit. An instant ago she froze; now she seemed to shatter into a thousand shards. Then she realised. The courier. He must be a German plant. There was no other explanation. No wonder he looked so relaxed, for he was in no danger at all. The soldiers knew; that's why they barely looked at his papers. And the Gestapo knew too. They were waiting for him to lead them from helper to helper, from safe house to safe house, all the way down the line, and every one of them would be rolled up and sent to concentration camps, and the line would die and the route over the Pyrenees would be closed for ever, and the airmen would be abandoned in a hostile country with no hope of return, no hope of resuming the fight, and the decent people would have lost and the wicked and the cruel would have won.

Her fear turned to fury. In that instant she went from
frozen cold to raging heat. She had to phone. She ran to the
nearest cafe and bought a jeton. There was a number to ring,
one that should never be used unless absolutely and utterly
necessary. It would connect her to the only person who
knew the whole line, who might be able to catch the courier
before the next handover. The phone rang, one ring. Ninette
picked up.

* * *

When Jose saw Parcel 42's head bobbing above the parapet
of the church tower it took him back to that night at Tante
Marie's. He'd never seen such a beanpole of a man. Would he
ever be able to bend low enough to run beneath the sweeping
searchlights? And how was he going to squeeze into the cave
on the border?

So Jose had looked a question at Ninette – Do I have to
take him? Is it worth the risk to the others, to you and me? In
return she gave him a look of disbelief. He sighed. He needn't
have bothered to ask. When did Ninette ever refuse to help a
parcel, in fact refuse to help anyone escaping the Nazis, even
Jews? It would get her caught one day, he knew it: she knew it
too, of course. It was bound to happen. Sooner or later she'd
be betrayed, but in the meantime she would save as many
as she could. Jose supposed he would go on until then too,
but it was easier for him, much easier, because he'd never be
caught. No one knew the mountains like he did. Even the
shepherds wouldn't find him if he didn't want them to.

Anyway, they couldn't go, not on a night like this. The
weather was terrible and it was going to get worse if he was

any judge of it. He'd be able to follow the path, just, but the first shelter was three hours away and by then the heavy rain in the valley would have soaked them all to the skin and the cold would freeze them to the bone. How far could they be expected to go in these conditions – a few miles and a thousand feet a night? Hardly more, and at that rate it would take them four nights to safety. Too long. They wouldn't survive four nights – at least some of them wouldn't. The Jew didn't look as if he'd ever walked across a city, never mind the Pyrenees.

He shook his head. 'We have to wait.'

He could see Ninette calculating. It was difficult for her, he understood perfectly. No doubt there were others coming down the line and expected to arrive soon. Tante Marie couldn't cope with more than five at a time – where would they sleep, how was she going to feed them? So Ninette would have to get a message back up the line in time to stop the next packages. And even if the message got through alright, was there a safe house they could stay in for longer? The repercussions might go all the way back to Normandy, Belgium, even Holland. And changes in arrangements led to confusion and mistakes.

'Two days,' she said.

He nodded, turned and walked out into the night. Straight into the arms of those little bastards of the Milice in their stupid black uniforms. He hated them worse than the Nazis. Most of the Boche didn't have a choice; they obeyed orders or got shot. The Milice were enthusiasts, volunteering to betray their own countrymen, taking revenge for petty insults and imagined hurts, sneaking around doing the Germans' dirty work. He hated the Milice, every single nasty one of them.

If there had only been two men that night, he'd have picked them up and banged their mean little heads together and left them for dead. But there were three. They surrounded him. One of them pointed a gun.

'Who are you? What are you doing here?'

'I'm a shepherd. Up in the hills. I came down to find a doctor. I'm in agony in my bowel.'

And with that Jose bent double and howled with pain. Ninette would hear and she would understand that it meant trouble.

'You're a bloody Spaniard. Get back to your side of the border.' And with that he kicked out at Jose.

'We'll kick you back to Spain.'

One of them laughed, a high thin sound, and then all three of them started kicking him. Jose howled louder. They're egging each other on, he thought, showing each other how tough they are. There's no boundary they won't cross, no stopping place. They could kill me, cripple me for life, and they wouldn't care. Then, though he had never before been frightened of any man, he felt the warm trickle down his leg and the unmistakable smell of urine. More kicks and then his bowels opened. He couldn't have prevented it if he'd tried. He was ashamed and pleased at the same time. They might believe him.

One of them hit him on the head with something and he fell to the ground. They each stamped on his abdomen as they left him there, and then went and banged on the door of Tante Marie's house. Jose knew that by then the parcels would have got through the hole behind the cupboard and into the grave in the orchard. They'd be alright. But Ninette would have to find another guide for them. He couldn't be seen here again for a while. In almost three years, it was the only time he would not be able to guide one of Ninette's groups. Limping away before they came back, he grieved the loss.

* * *

Genevieve knew that he was going to be at the reunion. Less than a year after the end of the war, he had written to ask if he could visit the farm. She had refused. She was trying to forget the horrors of the occupation, and she had a new boyfriend who had no idea she had been in the Resistance, so how could she explain a tall English stranger? Also she knew her parents had come to love him and had wanted him to stay on in spite of the risk, and they would try to persuade him to stay all over again. So no, it would be too much of a disruption. He wrote again saying he did not want to cause her any difficulty, but he did want to thank her properly and in person, to see the farm again and to pay his respects to her parents. She refused, knowing that he would not persist a second time.

But when her parents died she found herself telling the local priest that she wondered if she had done right, that it might have been a consolation to them to have his presence and his gratitude. 'Perhaps,' he had said, 'but never mind the dead, what about the living? I am not sure it is good for you to try to forget those times. You can never forget, and nor should you. You were doing Christ's work. Anyway, plenty of people here knew you were sheltering him but kept quiet about it, and that was dangerous enough in itself, as you well know.' He thought for a moment, then added, 'I suggest that the Mayor and I together, on behalf of France and the Church, invite him to come amongst us again and that we have a grand dinner with speeches and toasts, then his thanks to you will be in that context. He can stay with me.'

She said she'd think about it. And when she did she realised how reluctant she was to face the only person in the world who knew the worst of her. No one else would ever understand that she couldn't accept public praise for what she had done for him, and for others after him, for it had been in order to expiate her sin.

It had all got out of hand; in so many ways it had all got out of hand. She had taken him in on the understanding that it would be for one day only and that the next night she would take him to the crossroads in the wood at La Guelle where he would be collected. But whoever was supposed to come for him didn't turn up – not that night nor on any of the next three. So he stayed while she waited for instructions. The days turned into weeks and the weeks into months and still she waited. They seemed to have forgotten about him. The farm was remote and she kept him well hidden; also he did some of the heavy work, which was welcome, of course, especially when all the able young men were prisoners of war or slaves in Germany.

Gradually they had relaxed. He started to eat meals with them and to sleep in the house instead of behind a stall in the stable. He learnt French and they began to talk properly, to make each other laugh and to share their hopes for life after the war. In time he became one of the family, so it was a shock when he told her one day that he would have to leave. He explained that he loved being with them, with her, but that he had to get back. There weren't enough pilots and it took a long time to train a new one. So every one of them who made it home to fly again was a small help to the war effort and a small defeat for the Nazis. What's more, anyone who managed to return gave heart to the other airmen, showing them that it was possible to survive being shot down and that there were people in France who would help them get home.

She tried to dissuade him but she knew he was right. She said she'd make contact with the Resistance for him and in the meantime she would teach him to look like a Frenchman, or at least a bit less like an Englishman. So he changed his posture, easing the stiffness in his back to a slouch, and he learned to walk with loose knees and feet splayed out. He spoke with head forward, looking at his own feet rather than the other person's eyes, and although he had never smoked he developed the knack of having a half-finished cigarette hanging from his lower lip. After three days she said he would do; he could go.

And it was on that night that she woke to hear a strange sound. At first she thought it was an animal in pain, some distance away, then she realised it was in the house. She got up. It was coming from his room. She lit a candle and pushed open the door to find him, the tallest and most upright of men, lying curled up like a doormouse and wailing into the blankets which he had stuffed into his mouth. He turned his face up towards her and she saw two enormous eyes, much bigger than his eyes, white all around the pupils, like a bullock the moment his throat was cut.

She sat down and put a hand on his shoulder. Gradually the wailing calmed. She waited. Finally he stretched out and said, 'I am so sorry.'

She shook her head. 'What is it?'

He made no reply.

'I insist,' she said. 'You owe me that much.'

It took all his strength but he told her. It was that if the Gestapo caught and tortured him, he would break and betray her and all the others who had helped him. The thought of all those kind and generous people, the people he admired, respected, loved, the thought of them being killed or sent to the camps, and because of him – and it happening to her – well, it was unbearable. It had haunted him day and night, and now he was about to leave it had overwhelmed him.

He was so ashamed of himself, ashamed that he had already put so many people at risk and that he didn't have the courage to go out there and face what each and every one of them had already faced on his behalf. More, what she had faced without breaking down as he had broken down. He did not know if he could live with himself.

It was a long night. By the end of it, and to try to help him feel less alone, she had told him her deepest shame, the thing she had done which would be a stain on her for the rest of her life. They had clung to each other in shared misery and by the end of the night they had made a plan. He would not go down the line any further, putting more people at risk. Instead she would get him a man's bicycle and he would ride on his own to Spain. A hundred and fifty miles. He could do it in three nights.

He set off in his workman's clothes. She kept the ridiculous suit.

The two gendarmes stopped him near Prades. His papers made no sense at all, and in any case he didn't have the ones he needed for the zone so near the border. They handcuffed him, threw his bicycle in the ditch and put him in the car. Lucien dropped Georges off at home – they took it in turns – and then said to Parcel 42, 'English? Escape? OK,' and gave him the thumbs-up. He took him all the way to Tante Mathilde's house, just like a taxi.

★ ★ ★

On the last night the five of them huddled together for warmth in a small cave less than a mile from the border. He was so tall that he had to squeeze in backwards and leave his legs lying outside.

Ninette giggled at the sight. 'You can't leave them there,' she said, 'they'll freeze to death.'

'Where do you suggest I put them?'

'Can't you bend over and bring them in underneath you?'

'Madam, I am an Englishman not a contortionist.'

Ninette giggled again. 'You must keep moving them, seriously.'

He lifted them in the air and pedalled.

'Stop it, stop it. It is not completely dark yet.'

'I'm sorry.'

She slid out of the cave, wriggled away on her belly and returned with handfuls of bracken which she packed round his legs. Then she slithered off again and added another layer. When she lay back down beside him he saw that all the front of her coat was dirty and wet. He was filled with remorse. He only had a short distance to go but she had to walk all the way back over the Pyrenees, on her own, through the mud and the snow, a journey which had already exhausted all of the men.

'When you get back? Can you rest?'

'Depends.'

He understood. It depended on whether there were more parcels to be escorted over the mountains, more houses to be found where they could stay, more messages to get back up the line in order to regulate the flow. He wondered, as he had wondered before, how she kept going, how she managed to live on constant alert, always looking for the smallest sign that a place was not safe or that a person was not to be trusted. And she had taken over from Jose the guide at a moment's notice.

'You are running the whole line, aren't you?'

She had never admitted it to anyone – perhaps she felt that if she did so once, it would be harder to deny later, when she was in the hands of the torturers.

'What can I do to help?'

He could feel her shrug her shoulders.

She was right, of course. Even offering was practically an insult.

They fell silent. Behind them the others fell asleep. Some time later he started to shake.

'Are you cold?' she whispered. 'You could take my coat.'

'It's not that; it is fear. It gets me like this occasionally.'

'I know.'

'You don't shake, though.'

'Shaking is strictly verboten when the Germans are examining your papers.'

He smiled. 'Indeed. It is a luxury. I've never quite thought of it like that before.' He paused again. 'May I ask you? How do you do it? When you are risking your life every day, how do you manage?'

She considered. Was she willing to talk about it? She had got so used to keeping secrets, to saying as little as possible, always the bare minimum; it was safer that way. And in any case she didn't have the energy to spare. On the other hand it was tempting. So many people needed her to be brave and confident that she could never let her guard down or confess to any weakness. It would be good to be able to do that, just once; it would be a luxury, to use his word. And he was as safe as anyone could possibly be. In a few hours time he would be gone and she would never see him again, even supposing they both survived the war, which was unlikely.

'It's a drug,' she said, 'the fear. I'm drugged. The woman who persuades the soldiers that our papers are correct, it is just that they haven't had the right orders; the one who gets information that a house is no longer safe and rushes round there hoping to arrive before the Gestapo and get the parcels out; the one who stays calm when there is a bang on the door in the middle of the night and keeps them waiting long enough to make sure the radio is hidden – that isn't me. It's a woman on drugs. I watch her, as if from outside. But as you say, it affects the whole body. It is not good. Not good really, to be on drugs, not for so long.'

'The drugs must wear off sometimes?'

A faint sigh. 'Not often. And when they do I feel tired. And small.'

He almost laughed at that – she couldn't have been more than five feet high. But then he realised what an admission it was.

'I feel much smaller than you,' he said.

'Only without your legs.'

'That's true. They've dropped off.'

A tiny giggle. He was so glad to hear her laugh.

'But that's not the worst,' she went on. 'The worry is worse. The fear drives me on but the worry...that drains me. I can't...'

He waited and then said, 'Go on.'

'...can't ever rest. There's always a blockage somewhere along the line so there are ten parcels in a house that can only cope with four – how to get enough food to them? – and just the sound of the toilet flushing too often is enough to arouse suspicion. Or information hasn't got through and there's a parcel sitting on a bench somewhere waiting for a courier who doesn't know he's supposed to be there, or who has been caught, and I have to find a replacement fast. Or there's some idiot – some of the parcels are idiots – who has insisted on going for a walk from a safe house in the daytime so everyone can see there is a stranger there. Or Jose falls into the arms of the Milice, so here I am away from everyone and everything for eight days with no idea what's going on back up the line and what I'll find when I get back. Oh, it sounds as if I'm complaining but I'm not. It's a war and I have to fight the enemy, here and in this way, but you asked me and…well…'

She stopped.

'Sleep now,' he said. 'Rest.'

'We have to leave at four, exactly.'

'I'll stay awake.'

He woke her at ten to four and they all crawled out of the cave. But when he came to stand up he found he couldn't. His legs had got so cold in the night that the circulation had practically stopped and his muscles didn't work.

'I'll take the others and come back for you. Put your legs in the cave and rub them.' And she was off. When she got back he was asleep and he barely woke as she pulled him out of the cave by his armpits, head first.

She watched him as he waded through the river and timed his run across the border road to safety. For the first time she was tempted to go too, but she bent to drink from a spring and then turned back and upwards.

8

Kidneys

Twins

HETTIE AND FLO WERE IDENTICAL TWINS, strongly built and bony with coarse sandy hair which stood out from their ears in a thick bob. They had the same handwriting and the same voice with the same intonations, so those who had known them all their lives could barely tell them apart. When they were girls their father often credited one with what the other had done or blamed the innocent child for some misdemeanour – which enraged them both. At the age of fifty-eight, the same lines and wrinkles were beginning to appear around their eyes and mouth.

Hettie was the elder by four and a half minutes, a seemingly insignificant difference but one which might as well have been four and a half years as far as they were concerned. For Flo admired her sister, adopted her opinions and had the habit of obedience to her wishes, all of which Hettie took as her due. And it was true that Hettie looked smarter, had more friends and was generally more successful in her work, so that what started out as a shared assumption gradually became the way the world saw them too.

When they were three years old their father, on a whim, bought a wooden bungalow overlooking Broscombe Bay. He was walking along the cliff path one day when he came across it lying in a sheltered spot below the sessile oaks, just where the cart track ran from the village down the coombe to the sea. The For Sale sign was weather-beaten and the verandah looked dangerously askew, but it reminded him of the house in Simla, also a wooden bungalow with a verandah and an enormous view, where he had been so happy as a child. He always said that his impulse had been to give his children something he had loved, but in his heart of hearts he knew he wanted it for himself, His wife, for whom the house had no special significance, thought that the beauty of the land and the delights of the beach below were barely compensations for the permanently damp bedclothes, the smell of the primus stove, the walk to the spring to collect water, the earth toilet and the long journey on the bus to the nearest town to do her shopping.

For the twins, however, it was paradise. Paradise on their first visit and paradise ever after. It was a source of constant joy to them that they knew every animal track in the valley, every lapwing's nest on the clifftops and every rockpool on the beach. They knew where the watercress grew and the crabs hid, where chanterelles came up in late summer and which eddy collected the best driftwood. From the call of the gulls below they knew the exact direction of the wind and from the sound of the waves breaking on the beach the exact moment the tide turned. It was where they had each started to discover the wonders of the sea and shore which became their passion and which would occupy them for the rest of their lives. Together they collected shells and classified them; together they sat on the rock shelf and threw sticks into the sea to see which way the current was flowing; together they marked the limit of the highest and lowest tides; together they saw the sea turn silver as a shoal of mackerel swam into the bay and then flipped over to swim out again.

Although they loved it equally, they found as they grew older that their interests started to diverge. They knew, of course, that high tide was not at the same time each day, but it was Hettie who wanted to know why it was fifty minutes later, and why the fortnightly high and low tides came at the same time of day. Her father bought her a book but its explanations just led to more questions: 'If the moon and sun combined pull the water up and down, why don't they pull the land up and down too?' she demanded. 'Don't be silly, dear,' said her mother. When Hettie later discovered that it did, and worked out by how much, her mother still didn't believe her.

Nor was she satisfied with the tide tables – data at Plymouth was much too inaccurate – so she started to compile her own. As she added more and more information to the basic times and heights of the tide, she discovered all sorts of other correlations. 'The tide is always higher when the weather is awful,' she announced at dinner one day. 'I doubt it,' said her father, but it turned out she was right about that too. Then she realised that as high tide was a little later all the way up the coast to Scotland there must be a kind of giant wave flowing north. For her school maths project she calculated that the distance between the peak of each wave must be 362.5 miles; it took her teacher quite a long time to work it out and arrive at the same figure.

But while Hettie's curiosity took her away to the movement of the heavens and the oceans, Flo's was satisfied by the life on her own small beach, the limpets and starfish, the mussels and clams, the cuttlefish and sea anemones, the sea sorrel and bladderwrack, the periwinkles and crabs, and the jellyfish which were washed up at especially high spring tides. She studied them, she drew them and she collected them. But to her surprise the moment she later called her epiphany happened not on the beach but when she was in the middle of London.

On day, when she was eight years old, she had taken her favourite shells back to the family's London house and arranged them on a low table in her bedroom. That night she was woken by a scrabbling sound. At first she thought it must be mice in the roof but as she lay awake listening she suddenly knew it was in the room. Turning on the light, she saw that one of her shells was moving. And out if it protruded a long and spiny leg. She was fascinated. She watched as more legs appeared, then a claw, then eyes.

Gradually the legs shuffled the shell to the edge of the table. She was about to get out of bed to stop it falling when the creature eased itself over the corner with every appearance of deliberate care. And then walked around the underside of the table, still carrying the shell, moving two or three legs at a time while the others hung on over the top edge. She had never seen anything so wonderful in all her life.

She didn't go back to sleep that night. She ran an inch or two of water into the plug end of the bath – he must need water, mustn't he, if he lived in a sea shell? There was no seaweed in the house so she made do with some leaves from the rubber plant in the hall and put them in too, along with her other shells. Sand; she needed sand. The gardener kept his carrots in sand. She tiptoed downstairs, out into the dark garden and into the potting shed. She filled a flowerpot and as she came back through the kitchen door there was her mother looking fierce. 'Whatever are you doing, Flo? It's three o'clock in the morning.'

'Come. See.' Flo led her mother upstairs, hoping that the creature was still performing his upside-down trick. He was, but unexpectedly her mother was not entranced. She screamed, 'Take him out, take him away!' To her surprise, Flo found she was reluctant to pick him up, but she managed it and carried him, shell down (she didn't want him falling out onto the carpet), to the bathroom and put him in the bath with the sand.

'Not in the bath. I can't have that creature in my bath.' Her mother had followed her. By now her father had woken up and joined them. 'It's alright,' he said, 'we'll get him a proper aquarium in the morning.' Flo's heart leapt. It meant she could keep him. Her mother went back to bed muttering while the two of them sat on the floor and watched.

He seemed interested in his new home. First he made for the beach, still lugging his shell with him, dug himself a bit of a hole and settled into it. They thought he would stop there but he had only just started. As soon as he had made sure of his bed he set off to explore his new world. First he came across the rubber plant leaf, turned it over a few times, sat on it, and then seemed to decide he had exhausted its possibilities. By contrast he was captivated by the first shell he came to. He walked round and round it, tapping it with his legs. Quite quickly he abandoned the shell he was wearing and started to move in. It was a bit smaller than the old one so it was quite a job. But he soon he abandoned that one too and set off again.

When Hettie woke up and joined them he was grappling with the plug chain. She pretended to be interested but Flo could see she wasn't, not really. It was the first time they had not shared something, not been of one mind. So in the midst of her joy she felt a stab – did this mean her sister would be lost to her? And how would she manage without her?

But nothing more came between them. They went to the same university where they shared a flat and they still spent all their holidays in Broscombe. After they graduated they both stayed on to do research. Hettie studied the volcanos of the Atlantic islands. She thought that even a small eruption could set off a tsunami, and calculated that under certain quite common atmospheric conditions it could be between four and five metres high when it reached the south and west coast of Britain, enough to cause enormous devastation. 'Well, we haven't had one yet,' said her mother, 'not even four or five inches.'

Flo got a job as a very junior research assistant monitoring the populations of intertidal oysters. One day she read a paper written by an American professor who also had an interest in these oysters. He had taken some of them from a Connecticut shoreline to his lab at the University of Chicago so he could observe their behaviour more closely. He discovered that after a while they changed their feeding rhythm. They continued to open and shut in unison, and with unvarying regularity, but he couldn't understand their timing; what tune were they dancing to? It wasn't the tides in Connecticut where they had come from, nor anywhere else – he had checked all the tide tables he could find and there was no correlation. What was the explanation for this extraordinary behaviour?

Flo knew at once. Never mind that they were in glass boxes in a university building; never mind that Chicago had no tides. Given the tide times on both the east and west coasts of America at the same latitude, the oysters had worked out when high tide in Chicago ought to be. The Professor took

Flo's suggestion seriously and moved them to Alberquerque, New Mexico. And after a while the oysters adjusted their timing to high tide in the high desert. Flo was ecstatic. She just knew their behaviour would make sense.

'But it's not a proper tide,' said Hettie, 'so it doesn't really count, does it?'

Over the years Hettie became internationally famous for her work and she travelled the world lecturing to scientific bodies and advising port and harbour authorities. When governments planned tidal barrages they came to Hettie to find out the optimum height they would need to be and the maximum force they would have withstand. There were those who criticised her for exaggerating the risks and demanding over-engineered solutions; to which she always replied that there was no point in protecting a major city from minor inconvenience if it was devastated by flood waters a year or two later. And, she would go on, quite apart from the unimaginable cost, did any of her critics think what it would be like to come out of your front door and face a five-foot tidal wave coming down the street towards you?

Flo's work, though it never achieved anything like the same degree of recognition, was influential in its way too. She had lovingly monitored the marine life on Broscombe beach for nearly fifty years, noting the extent of the six kinds of seaweeds which grew there, the areas inhabited by barnacles which could not survive high tides, the competition for space among the crustaceans and gastropods, the populations of wading birds – in fact, year after year she painstakingly recorded the state of everything that lived in that strip of land between the highest and the lowest tides, that place which spoke, though she would never admit to such a grandiloquent notion, of the health of the whole planet. She did the work for its own sake but others used it. Hettie borrowed the data to calculate some of the effects of climate change on the Atlantic currents, and thanks to Flo's observations a marine biologist found an explanation for a new and virulent strain of fish disease.

It was the day after their fifty-eighth birthday and they were walking together on the beach when Hettie told Flo that she had been diagnosed with cancer. Flo's hands flew to the very top of her chest. 'Oh my love,' she said, 'oh my love.'

'Treatment starts week. Mr Collins, quite a young man but he's doing the most up-to-date research. I wanted a scientist not a clinician. I checked on the statistics, of course, and they look good.'

Hettie paused, clearly waiting to be asked about survival rates, but Flo couldn't think of anything to say to that. Instead, she reached out her hand and tucked it under Hettie's arm. Flo hadn't expected a response of softness or yielding, though it would have been a comfort.

'What can I do?'

'Nothing. There's nothing to do. I'll carry on as usual. There may be some days after the treatment when I'll feel unwell but I can just work at home then.'

'I could look after you.'

'I don't want looking after, and anyway I won't need it. I'm going to fight this thing and I'm going to beat it.'

Flo knew she ought to feel pleased that Hettie was so determined but she felt her heart sink. Was it a battle, truly? Was it a war? She saw armies clashing, cells lying like bodies sprawled in death; she saw the exhaustion of the conquerers even in their victory and watched as the defeated forces rallied more troops to renew the onslaught.

Hettie broke the silence. 'Aren't you going to ask me where it is?'

'Sorry, of course,' she said, though she couldn't see it mattered. 'I was just thinking.'

'Localised Hodgkin's. Interesting man actually.'

'Who?'

'Hodgkin. Thomas Hodgkin. He dissected cadavers and noticed a common enlargement of the lymph glands in a number of them. Everyone else assumed it was syphilis or tuberculosis, but he realised it wasn't, that it was different. Wonderful, don't you think? To look at something that lots of people had seen before but to see it afresh. He saw a new disease – well, actually a new version of an old disease. I like that.'

Flo was not really surprised for she knew her sister of old. But she couldn't help wondering if there was real fear underneath. She certainly felt it herself. But then, she reflected, if it were her cancer, she would want to stand still, to not move from this beach, this house, this valley, and to wait and watch as it washed over her, to lose herself in the fascinated observation of the changes in her body. It would be remarkable to see a natural process distorted, subverted, out of control, and to notice her own reactions to each stage of the progression; there would be so much to learn. But Hettie was different. Hettie's attention would be turned away from her own experience and outwards into the world of experiments and research papers, of chemistry and pharmacology. Her determination would also be to understand – they did have that in common – but it would overlook her own unique predicament. In fact, thought Flo, she probably wouldn't believe there was such a thing.

But Hettie had to be supported, whatever her choice. That was the point. The two of them had been together since before they were born and they had to stick together. Flo vowed to herself that she would not give her advice, would not try to persuade her to do anything differently and would not criticise or undermine her decisions.

She thought Hettie would like it if she asked about the treatment.

'Radiotherapy. By far the best bet for localised Hodgkins,' said Hettie.

'What's radiotherapy?'

'Basically X-rays. High-powered X-rays, very focussed. They burn the cancer cells to death.'

'With heat, Hettie? Surely not heat.' The words just burst out of her. She had broken her vow, she realised, only moments after making it.

'Of course. What do you think? That they can just wash them off with water?'

'I'm so sorry,' said Flo. 'Silly of me. I don't know what I was thinking.' Except that actually it was more or less what she did think. Oh, it was ridiculous of her to oppose the knowledge and experience of the doctors, she knew that, but some deep instinct held that heat was bad and water was good.

'It's just surgery really. Think of it as surgery but done with beams instead of a knife. I'm lucky. The technology is extraordinary these days, precisely targeted to kill the mutant cells.'

Flo knew that Hettie was trying to reassure her, but she was making it worse. It was just so hard to believe that it would be good for her to have intense beams, which the human body had never encountered before, and to which it would have no defence whatever, penetrating and destroying a part of her.

And what about all the other cells, the healthy ones, the ones Hettie needed, not least to recover – would they survive? Could the technology really be so discriminating? And what would it be like to be powerless as all this happened, to rely completely on the state of knowledge of Mr Collins, a man you'd hardly met and who might have all kinds of prejudices and blind spots, who might even be wildly over-confident?

It was like when they were children and their mother used to read aloud to them and the two of them used to drive her mad by constantly asking questions which pointed out all the holes in the story she was reading, and she would always say, 'Oh, for heaven's sake, don't ask so many questions, it's just a story.' Well, my questions are like that, thought Flo; they are pointing out the holes in the story. But Hettie wouldn't see it that way. She wouldn't think it was a story; she'd think it was science.

'I've asked all the questions, as you can imagine,' said Hettie, 'and I am quite satisfied with the answers.'

Flo just managed to stop herself saying that Hettie had certainly not asked all the questions; in fact she hadn't asked the biggest question of all – Why had she got it? And then, as she lay awake in the middle of the night, she realised that there was an equally big question she had not asked herself – Why haven't I got it? After all, she reasoned, we are identical twins with exactly the same genes organised in exactly the same way, and we have led very similar lives, neither of us smoking, for example. When we were ill as children we both had the same illnesses at the same time; so perhaps, or even surely, I have cancer too.

Flo supposed she could take whatever tests Hettie had taken and find out, but she knew she was not going to. She imagined Hettie's life over the next few years; days and days

spent sitting in airless, windowless hospital waiting rooms, all
plastic and metal, hard and bright; submitting to the constant
invasion of tests and treatments; getting to like some nurses
and not others and hoping each time that she would get one
of the ones she liked; seeing figures on a graph that told
her she was doing better, or worse, as if the figures were
the reality; having her hopes raised by this result or dashed
by that; suffering from the side effects of the treatment and
having to believe that feeling worse was a good thing and a
necessary stage on the road to recovery; and fighting, all the
time fighting – that would be exhausting in itself, wouldn't it,
and dispiriting too?

Well, it was not her way. She would not contemplate
changing her life to do the things she didn't want to do instead
of the things she did. And when it came to an end she hoped,
she trusted, that she would have the grace to leave it with
some dignity, for just as it had been given to her so it would
be taken away, and it seemed to her a bit ungrateful to object
– like being a spoilt child who makes a fuss when she is told to
go to bed at a perfectly reasonable time.

She stretched out in bed, feeling the arch of her back,
the strength of her thighs, the tightness in her shoulders,
the dryness of her skin against the sheets and the size of her
hands which suddenly felt huge, like on a skeleton. It was
good to pay attention to these things; in fact she was not sure
she'd ever done it before, and certainly not in a systematic
way. For she had never really thought of her body as herself,
as Florence, the biologist, the unrequited lover, the sister, the
woman who had spent her life on Broscombe beach. Perhaps
her miscarriage hadn't helped.

No, it was her brain that was her, thoughts and ideas, and
perhaps emotions too now she thought of it, and her body was

simply what carried it all around. It was a vehicle – she smiled
at the notion – though not a car which was too small, nor a
lorry which was too big, but, but…a pick-up truck. A delightful
image; she liked it. That's what it was, a pick-up truck. Well,
she would get to know this pick-up truck and maybe it was
her after all in the same way as her brain was her. And perhaps
it was ageing, and dying, at the same rate as her brain, so
they could stay together and leave together. Hettie's brain,
on the other hand, would be in armed combat with her body
for the rest of her life, and Flo didn't envy her that.

What would she miss most? The beach, naturally, which
was almost as much a home to her as to all the multitude of
species which lived there too. A small world in the opinion
of many of her colleagues, but it was plenty big enough
for her; after all, no one could ever know it entirely, nor
understand it fully. She wouldn't miss Hettie because Hettie
would outlive her, and Hettie wouldn't miss her because she'd
be too busy dying.

Regrets? None at all, except, only a slight amendment,
she did wish she'd studied octopuses properly. What endlessly
inventive creatures they are, she thought. It pleased her that,
like her hermit crab from long ago in her child's bedroom
in London, they would colonise shells and live in them, but
even more she loved that they can change their appearance
at will, going from pale to dark, or vice versa, and even better
that they can have one half dark and the other light. She'd
watched them go the exact colour and texture of a rock they
are lying on and apparently, though she had never seen it,
they can even go striped. She couldn't imagine what use that
could possibly be, so she decided that they must do it for fun,
like the gardens they make in front of the places they live.
They can walk on tiptoes or become jet-propelled, moving

at high speed with tentacles trailing behind. They have blue blood and three hearts. Their suckers stick to everything like the strongest glue but don't stick on themselves and she had always wondered how they do that. They can squirt out a huge cloud of ink and depart behind it so you can't see which way they've gone. They can deflate themselves and squeeze through the tiniest of holes and, possibly best of all in Flo's opinion, if you put them in a tank they can usually work out how to dismantle it, and then do so and escape.

It didn't matter how long she had left. She wanted to study octopuses, not in tanks and aquariums, but in their natural habitat. She sat up in bed, excited. She was going to have to have to give up her job and learn to dive; she was going to have to go and live in Greece where octopuses were common.

In the next year there was barely a day when Flo did not spend some time underwater at Areopoli. It was wonderful. She could hardly believe that in all those years on Broscombe beach she had never thought of diving. As she slipped beneath the surface she could leave everything behind, all thoughts of Hettie's illness, her own, all the irritations and the sufferings of normal life, and float into a timeless world. The joy of being practically weightless, of having a body which surprised her by seeming neither awkward nor ungainly, was a revelation. The slightest twitch of a hand or foot, hardly more than thought of a movement really, would turn her this way or that, roll her over and over, or twist her gaze to where she wanted it to fall. My body might be starting to break down and be consumed by the disease, she thought, but at least I am inhabiting it for the first time in my life. Relishing it actually.

The local fishermen told her that there weren't nearly as many octopuses as there used to be. The sea had been overfished and was becoming polluted so it no longer supported the diversity of life they had known as children. She paid them not to catch octopuses locally, nor the crabs which formed their most common diet, and she became known locally as the madwoman – who else would pay fishermen not to work? In time she marked out an area to be protected where they knew she would be underwater each day and which they ended up patrolling to make sure that boats from other villages did not take advantage. They made more money from her than they would have done from fishing, and in any event, they reasoned, she wouldn't stay for long and the area would provide rich pickings when she was gone.

From time to time she heard from Hettie. It turned out that the radiation hadn't worked; apparently the lymphoma wasn't local enough after all and it had spread. But she said that Flo wasn't to worry because there was a remarkable new procedure. The drugs that attacked the cancer cells affected healthy cells too, and particularly the ones deep in the bones which made blood; so they would be harvested and kept outside the body while the drugs killed all the cancer cells and then the healthy cells would be put back again. Hettie enthused about the brilliance of the notion, about the sophistication of the technology and the skill of Mr Collins and his dedicated team.

At this distance it all seemed unreal to Flo, like an airport thriller with an implausible plot, cardboard characters and a predictable ending. She told herself a very different story. For although she became bronzed and fit she was under no illusions. She was losing weight steadily, had little appetite and was increasingly aware of a pain which had started in her lower back but now seemed to wander about her body, affecting now her neck, now her hips, now her jaw. Some days it disappeared; on others it made it hard to get out of bed in the morning, though she always managed it in the end. That wasn't where she was going to die. One day she would lose strength underwater and simply not come up from a dive. She couldn't imagine a better ending.

When Hettie was informed that Flo had drowned she felt a wave of regret that she had not been there with her sister. But there was no body, hence no funeral, and in any case she was too unwell to travel. She lived for another few weeks in a hospital bed, still hoping for a remission, and it was only when she felt an overpowering thirst that her will started to give way. She was comforted by the thought that she had played her part in a noble search for a cure, and that by donating her body to science something of her would survive.

9

Pericardium

Opening the gate

JAMES SATTERTHWAITE WAS BORN IN 1634 AT Long Howe Colthouse, lived there all his life and slept and died in the same bed. If you had asked him why, he would have smiled and said it was the best place on earth – not that he had seen many others as the longest journey he ever made was to visit people in gaol in Lancaster, all of thirty miles away.

Like his father and grandfather before him he farmed twenty acres of good valley land by the lane towards Wray, and had a herd of sheep on the fells. Like them he was christened at St Thomas's in Hawkshead. But one day, at the age of eighteen, he fell in with a man walking along the lane towards Ambleside who told him that there was that of God in everyone and that he needed no priest to tell him what the Lord wanted of him; on the contrary, it was the prompting of love in his heart that was the leading of God. For James it was the plain truth and from that day on he never set foot in St Thomas's again. So on a Sunday, when his parents were at church, he invited people to sit with him in the parlour to wait on those promptings.

'Are you praying or what?' his father had asked.

'Not what you would call praying,' was the young man's reply, 'for there is no set form and no insincere babble. But certainly what we would call praying as we respond to an awareness of the living Christ.'

His father expected the boy would grow out of it.

But he was wrong. Within a year, the three or four who had first joined James in the parlour each Sunday had grown to almost twenty. For the parish priest it was beginning to look like a challenge to his authority; and besides there would surely be grave dangers to the spiritual health, not to mention the morality of the local community, if any untutored farm boy felt entitled to set up his own church. Still, he didn't want to be heavy-handed and call in the local magistrate, at least not yet, so he had a word with James's father and from then on the parlour was closed to them.

No one else had a room big enough so they met outside, in Frank Tyson's field, whatever the weather. Frank had never liked the priest, and anyway James had always been willing to give him a hand with jobs he wasn't strong enough to do any more. In summer they sat on two long benches in the shade of the beech trees, and in winter they huddled under one of the walls. In the long evenings of June, James would go up the fell and bring down stones to build up those walls so they would provide more protection from wind and rain.

The priest consulted the magistrate. It seemed that there was no illegality in people sitting outside provided there was no trespass. So the priest went to Frank Tyson, asking him to forbid them entry. Frank demanded to know if there was a law these days preventing a man making whatever use he wanted of his land, and if so, it was surely the end of property and of the England he knew and would defend to his dying breath. The priest withdrew, red-faced and angry. But Frank realised that he had only won a battle and he had no stomach for a war. He went to James and offered to sell him the field for a guinea, and it was purchased, not in James's name alone but in the names of all those who attended the meetings each Sunday.

The following years were hard. The next spring was exceptionally cold and summer came so late that they only got one cut of silage instead of two, not enough to feed all their animals through the winter. James had to slaughter cows, though it grieved him to do so. And the summer after was so wet that the hay rotted in the field before it could ripen. James's father went to the Earl of Lonsdale's steward and begged for a reduction in the rent, as did all the tenants in the area, and like them was refused. There were no savings to tide them over so the rest of the herd was sold. The old man had tended his cows, cared for them, milked them day in day out and worried about them on the rare occasions he was away from the farm for a day or two, and the loss killed him. The day James took them off to market in Kendal, he sat in his chair by the fire, refused all food and drink and was found there the next morning, slumped over, rigor having already set in.

James went to see the priest about the funeral. 'I'll bury him in holy ground and in full observance of all the rites of the Church, just as it should be and as he would have wished. He was a decent God-fearing man, your father,' said the priest. Then, 'You'll want it done nice and quiet; respectful?'

'Of course.'

'Well, in that case you'll do well to stay by the lych gate and come no further.'

'My own father's burial?'

'If you want no trouble.'

When he told his mother she wept for the first time since her husband had died. 'It would've broken his heart,' she said, 'his own son not in church to pay his respects.'

'I can pay them at the lych gate, mother. I can pay them anywhere.'

'Pay them in that field of yours then, and break it twice over.'

She only survived her husband for a few months and James was left alone in the farmhouse, the last in a long line of Satterthwaites.

The Sunday after her funeral he sat with his friends in Tyson's field, as everyone still called it, and he thought that it was plain daft to be outside now when there was no one to stop him using the parlour again. But he couldn't do it. He owed his father that much. Then he thought of using one of the barns, the lower one, at least when not lambing. It would be dry, if not warm. But that didn't seem right either. For one thing they deserved better, and for another it would look to the world as if they were hiding away. What they needed was a decent room, not one used for daily life with all its clutter, but one reserved for worship. Not like St Thomas's, no tower or steeple, in fact no nave or aisle, no lectern or communion rail, not even a cross come to that, for Jesus was in their hearts or not present at all. A good room, though, the ceiling higher than the parlour, the windows taller, the walls panelled. A sanctuary of quiet which would lift the spirits of all who attended there.

And then James remembered St Francis and how he had gone from house to house asking not for money but for stones with which to build his chapel. Well, he could do the same without the bother of begging, for there were stones aplenty to be had for the price of a little sweat. So at the end of meeting one late summer's day he paced out the building. Better too big than too small; you only do it once. And it would bring more people to join them, he was sure of that: those who would be glad to sit in such a handsome place to feel the presence of the Lord. And in hundred years, or even two, there might be more people meeting for worship here than in St Thomas's. He wouldn't say that to anyone for they might think him presumptuous, but all the same it cheered him as he worked.

It took him two years to lay out the foundations, for they were the biggest and heaviest stones of all. Bringing them down from the fell was hard work but rough hewing them was harder still. A few friends offered to help but he always refused. It was his idea, his task and his offering, and he had set his heart on having it as he had seen it that day, sitting under the wall in the soft September light. Anyway, none of them really understood. For example, right from the start they asked why he had set the building almost in the centre of the field and back from the lane instead of in the corner where he could have made use of two of the existing walls. 'Because of the journey inward,' he replied, 'and outward, of course.' The wall along the lane was going to be at least six feet high with a doorway right in the centre. Then to come in through that door would be to leave the everyday world behind and enter a quiet and sheltered space where people could ready themselves to turn towards the Lord. After that, the door of the Meeting House would then be a second, inner gateway, leading them to the sanctuary within.

Another year and the walls were barely two feet high. It became know locally as Satterthwaite's folly, and even those who met in the field each week doubted it would ever be finished. 'We'll be long gone before you're done,' said June Birkin, 'and chances are you will be too.'

'We're no more than a few,' James replied. 'But think of those as come after. How many will worship here all through a hundred years, two hundred, more? Thousands. It's for them more than us. And for someone who don't count time like you and me.'

Roger Wetherby, the stonemason, came to look one day and spent an hour or more examining every stone and joint. 'No so bad,' he said at the end, a man of few words. Then, 'Bottom step of stair's not right.' James looked at it.

'You want limestone.'

'Maybe so, but there's none round here to gather.'

Two weeks later Roger's cart appeared in the lane with seven limestone slabs, dressed and shaped.

James was speechless.

'But, but...' He wanted to say that Roger was a churchgoer, that it was too generous a gift, that he would never be able to repay, that he couldn't accept, but the words wouldn't come out right.

'Do the job proper,' was Roger's only comment.

So James built the staircase next, before the walls were much above waist height. It did look strange, sticking out from the porch and ending in the sky. People couldn't believe it.

'You want an upstairs?' they said, as if he was mad.

'Gallery,' he smiled at them.

'Alright, gallery. But what for?'

'For folks who are late. They'll not disturb the meeting that way.'

James was a good-looking young man and his land was a pleasure to behold, well farmed and well maintained, so there were plenty of local girls who widened their eyes at him.

He nodded to them politely as they happened to walk back and forth along the lane past the fields where he was working on a summer's day, but he took no trouble to come over to the gate and pass the time with them. Faith and Charity Denton who came to meeting with their parents had long given up trying to impress him, though Mary Thwaite prayed regularly that he would take notice of her.

He was twenty-eight, and the Meeting House walls were almost up to his waist, when he was called from the fields one day by Bert Langton with the news that there were five strangers waiting for him at his farmhouse door. When he arrived they were sitting in the porch. He was struck by the fact that there was no chatter between them and it almost looked as if they were meeting for worship, right there and then on a Tuesday afternoon. Nor did there seem to be any deference offered or accepted, although the distinctions of rank were clear.

The first to greet him was a gentlewoman, but by the looks of them the elderly man and one of the girls were servants. As for the other two, he took them to be the gentlewoman's daughters, though it turned out that one was a niece. And it was the niece whose sweet nature shone out at him with a lovely openness so different from the bold looks or silly simperings of the local girls that he felt a catch in his heart.

James greeted them, showed them into the parlour, gave them water from his best jug and was about to ask what they wanted of him when the lady spoke.

'We are travelling to Carlisle to the aid of friends who are in gaol there, and would be glad of your hospitality for the night.'

She must have seen the expression on James's face for she continued, 'One room will suffice for us women. William will be glad of the straw in your barn. Payment will be made, naturally, for any nourishment you are able to provide.' But she misunderstood him. He had rooms to spare, hams in the chimney and cheese and bread in the larder to which she and her party were welcome; what surprised him was that a woman of her kind would have friends in gaol. And Carlisle! That was more than forty miles away, over the fells too, and there were no horses nor any coach, so they must be on foot, all the way, with only one old man to protect them and he not one to deter a rogue of settled intent.

They set off the next day and he accompanied them to show them the short way to Ambleside. When they arrived in the centre of the town the niece stood up on the steps of the church and started to call on all those passing by to cease from the teachings of men but to hearken to the light of Christ within. James motioned her to come down; there could be trouble. She took no notice and continued, saying that she had come to bear witness to His name and to declare the gospel of the living Lord. It didn't take long before people started jeering, and not much longer before stones were thrown. One hit her on the side of her head. James jumped up on the wall and pulled her away, shielding her from the crowd that had gathered. They all made their escape along the bridleway under Loughrigg.

At the stepping stones she stopped and said, 'Do you not agree with my words?'

'Of course.'

'Then why stop me from speaking them?'

'Because of the crowd. Because I feared for you, for your safety.'

'It is more important, surely, for the truth to prevail?'

'At the price of harm to you?'

'And whose choice is that?'

He bowed his head. 'I cannot argue with you. I did not want you to be hurt. I wanted to protect you.'

'Then do so. Accompany me.'

'To Carlisle?' He could hardly believe it.

She laughed.

'Carlisle is not far,' she said. 'Carlisle or London, Ireland or the Americas. Who knows where the Lord will call?'

'But the farm, the Meeting House…'

'Leave them. Leave it all and walk in obedience to the Lord. His goodness will accompany you everywhere.'

'No. No. It would be the act of a fool.'

'Then be a fool for Christ.' She smiled. 'And perhaps you will thereby become wise.'

He shook his head. 'No.'

One summer's evening, a few years later, James came in from the fields and there in the porch was the woman who had walked away from him under Loughrigg. She looked tired, older. 'Will you stay?' he asked. '

'A little while,' she replied. 'To recover my strength.'

In the daytime she would sit in the orchard reading and resting and in the evening he would light a fire in the parlour; he had never before had one in summer but she loved the warmth of it. Then she would tell him stories of her travels. 'Oxford was the worst. We were beaten and left for dead in the main street, then they came back the next day and found us lying there, unable to move, so they dragged us to the prison. But in spite of all we rejoiced in the Glory that was there revealed to many.' There was no reproach in her voice but James felt it in himself.

On the Sunday after her arrival she went with him to Tyson's field to join with those who gathered there each week and after sitting in silence for some while she got to her feet and ministered. It reminded James of the man he had met in the lane. As before, it was hard to believe that a frail human body could command such power and astonishing to see how a person could be so transparent that the words of the Lord could come through unmuddied by her own desires or dislikes. He saw his friends and neighbours look at her with awe. Then their eyes would slide across to him with a question – are they wed, in deed if not in form?

So that evening, by the fire, he asked her to marry him. She replied immediately. 'We each have the work we have been called to do. Yours is here with the farm and the Meeting House. I know that now. And mine is away, spreading the word of the Lord wherever he leads me to do so. Any marriage, for you or for me, must encompass our work.' At the time he took it as a refusal, hearing her say that he could not go and she could not stay, and only years later did he understand that she was offering a different kind of marriage. She would not be a farmer's wife nor bear his children, but she would commit to him, return to him and share his life in the spirit. He had not grasped her meaning because a marriage of that kind was beyond his imagining then.

As she left to go, she turned to him and told him that his Meeting House would be a beacon to all friends and a model for the future. 'Some of us will still need to travel and preach abroad, but many, many more will need to meet in quiet and listen for the still small voice within. Following the guidance of that voice will change them, change the world they live in, and in the end it will change the world beyond – further than Carlisle indeed,' she teased him, 'even Carlisle. So your work is the same as my work, and I devoutly hope that it is given to me to do mine as well as you do yours.'

James carried on with renewed strength and the next time she arrived the walls were up to their full height and the roof beams were being prepared. The time after that she attended her first meeting sheltered from the elements. 'Wherever I go,' she told him, 'I tell friends of your Meeting House and give them sufficient description that they can copy it. By the time it is completed there will be twenty or more, all children of yours and all bearing their father's face.' By her next visit there was panelling inside and a dias for the elders.

That time she stayed longer and when she left he walked with her to Lancaster to bring food and comfort to friends who had been jailed there. She had been to prison countless times, and not always as a visitor, so the slam of the huge nailed gate closing behind them held no terrors for her. Nor was she oppressed by the utter darkness which closed over them as they were admitted to the cell where six friends lived with no fresh air, no warmth, no notion of day or night. After two hours the jailer returned and as the door swung open to a dank and dirty passageway James wept. She took his hand to comfort him but it was no comfort.

And, to his enormous surprise, as they were let out of the main gate he wept too. 'What is it?' he asked. She shook her head, unable to speak. It was the first time he had known her with no words. They parted at the bottom of the hill below the castle, she to Bristol and he back home.

Some years later a stranger came to the Meeting House one Sunday. At the end of worship James welcomed him and offered him food. 'You have given me food once before,' the stranger said, and seeing the surprise on James's face he added, 'though it was in the dark.' Then James understood.

They went back to the farmhouse and talked long into the night. The stranger complimented James on the simple beauty of the Meeting House and the atmosphere of peace within. 'I know that you planned and built it yourself. I don't know how you could have done it; all those months and years of labour, and all alone.'

'It was nothing compared to what you did,' James replied. 'I could hardly bear to be in that cell for two hours, and you were there how long?'

'Eighteen months, bar a day or two.'

'How did you survive?'

The stranger smiled. 'I was reminded of it when I came to meeting here today. It is rather like, don't you think?'

'I can see no comparison.'

'The outer gate from the lane which separates from the world. A step away from the busyness of daily life. Then the door of the Meeting House itself which leads to the inner sanctuary. And there in the silence, in the gathered silence of friends, the light of Christ shines forth and the grace of God descends. You know that. Well, in prison we had those same conditions for meeting for worship all day and every day. And we did not have to build the gaol with our bare hands first.'

'You are telling me I have built a prison?' James laughed. 'Not so. My gates can be opened and shut at will.'

'Indeed?'

'Yes, indeed.'

'But the gate and the door are always closed, except during meetings, and locked, are they not?'

'They are, but anyone can get the keys from me. And, of course, unlike your prison, no one is locked in.'

'Really?'

James knew that the man was saying something behind and beyond the natural meaning of his words, but he did not care to know what it was.

The conversation had unsettled him and James knew he would not sleep. So he went up on the fell by moonlight and sat under Middling Crag waiting for the dawn to break. In his mind was that visit to Lancaster goal and he thought of the woman who had left him there, as she had that first time under Loughrigg, and whom he had not seen since. And although she had returned many times between the two partings, he had a feeling that she would not come back again.

The stranger. He had known her. Did he have some news of her, some message? Were his words some kind of guidance? Was he suggesting that the gate onto the lane and even the door of the Meeting House itself should stay open and offer welcome to any who cared to come within? Of course, there were those who wished no good to him and to the congregation who worshipped there, but perhaps if they came in with mischief in their minds they might be affected by the peace within and leave with less trouble in their hearts. It might be indeed that they would be opened to the God within and that they would turn towards Him in joy.

James went down and unlocked the gate in the wall. It felt wonderful. But in the porch of the Meeting House itself, with its huge steel key in his hand, he hesitated. His breath became quick and shallow. He found that he was frightened. It felt as if he was opening himself to danger, to harm. Then an image of her came to him as she stood on the steps of the Church in Ambleside, preaching amidst a hail of abuse and standing firm as stones were hurled at her, and he knew that she had done so a thousand times and never flinched. And indeed that one day she had been killed by a similar mob, here or in Ireland or America, it didn't matter where, and that she would not have had it otherwise, and that was why she had not returned and why she had wept on the steps of Lancaster gaol. And so he turned the key in the lock, swung open the heavy door, and walked home.

10

Three Heater

Soft bamboo

SI PYO LIN TURNED TO HIS COMMANDING officer and said apologetically, 'Here you must take your shoes off, sir.' Colonel Hutchins removed his shoes, handed them to the young man and started up the first step in his stockinged feet. Si Pyo Lin darted after him. 'I am very sorry, sir. I did not make myself clear. No shoes or socks. Bare feet only.' Hardly breaking stride, Colonel Hutchins removed one sock and stuffed it in his pocket, then did the same with the other. Si Pyo Lin felt a wave of gratitude and affection for the man. Many of the Colonel's fellow officers, including those considerably junior to him, would have sworn at the request and only complied with an enormous show of reluctance, all the while making stupid jokes about the natives. And there were even some who would have refused and smirked while defiling this most holy of sites.

The Colonel was a big man in his fifties and it took him some effort to climb the two hundred and sixty steps to the pagoda, but once he had started up he maintained a steady pace all the way to the top. That's what Si Pyo Lin had come to admire – the steadiness. Once the Colonel embarked on a task he saw it through. Si Pyo Lin wanted to be like that, and he promised himself that when the British left he would try to live up to the Colonel's example.

It was early evening and people were starting to arrive after work, gathering to make their prostrations, to meditate in front of one of the golden Buddhas, and then to sit in clusters to chat and gossip. From time to time small children would detach themselves from the clusters, run around and then come back to throw themselves into the arms of their mothers. Colonel Hutchins approved of this combination of the ordinary and the holy, and rather wished that the Anglican services he was obliged to attend could have a bit more of both.

Si Pyo Lin, as he strolled along, one step behind the Colonel, was proud of his fellow countrymen. They looked up at the soldier in full uniform, the head of an army which had invaded their country, deposed their king and turned his palace into a barracks, and their glance was neither servile nor resentful. Instead it contained a simple acceptance. Si Pyo Lin wished that his older brother would take the same attitude. For Han Min, the British were simply oppressors intent on stealing the natural resources of Burma. While the younger brother was proud that its teak was furnishing the homes of Glasgow merchants and its oil was fuelling the factories of Birmingham, the older man saw it as an outrage. And far from admiring Si Pyo Lin's rise to a position in the administration of the country, as his parents had done, he judged it a treachery. 'Just wait till the British are gone,' he used to say, 'and you find yourself on the wrong side of history.'

Well, Si Pyo Lin couldn't see that there would be any less need for proper administration when the British had gone, nor that history would criticise those who had maintained good order and indexed records. But his brother's revolutionary zeal had no time for mundane administration, and, even if his charisma marked him out as a future leader, he would not be the one who paid attention to routine or efficiency. Si Pyo Lin supposed he would have to clear up Han Min's mess, as he always had done.

The Colonel turned to him. 'Why so may Buddhas? Are they different in some way?'

'Not different, not in this tradition, sir. It is a matter of devotion.'

The Colonel slapped his baton against his thigh and cleared his throat. Si Pyo Lin knew these as the signs that the Colonel wanted more information so he continued. 'A heart which recognises the gift of the Buddha's teaching wants to give a gift in return. It is an acknowledgment and an obeisance. Also...' Si Pyo Lin paused, wondering if he was about to overstep his position.

'Go on, man.'

'When it comes from the heart then it does not measure what is enough. It does not ration.'

Colonel Hutchins smiled. 'No Buddist quartermaster's stores?'

'No, sir.'

'The more the better, in fact?'

'Yes, sir.'

The Colonel considered. It certainly wasn't how he had been brought up nor how he had been trained as an officer. In fact, now he thought about it, he didn't think he'd ever given anyone more than enough. He was devoted to Enid, of course he was, but he had never bought her a present which, in his judgment, she did not need. He remembered once walking through a bazaar together when she had taken a fancy to a finely worked pair of leather gloves. Although she clearly wanted them, he had not got them for her because she already had a pair of leather gloves. Did that mean he wasn't really devoted? Was there a case for abundance?

Colonel Hutchins slapped his thigh and cleared his throat. 'Would you do this yourself, provide another Buddha here?'

'Not here, sir. But in my home village, yes. Once I have made sure my parents are provided for.'

Well, my parents are well provided for, thought Colonel Hutchins, so according to Si Pyo Lin's lights I should purchase a golden Buddha. He felt a sudden temptation to do so. He'd never tell anyone, of course. They'd say he'd gone native. Which would be true, he supposed. Except that they'd mean it as a bad thing while, at the moment, it seemed to him rather a good one. At any rate he'd much rather buy a statue of a man sitting quietly and smiling at the predicament of his fellow human beings than one of a man on a cross, being tortured to death. He sighed. Leaving Burma and retiring to Cheltenham or Tunbridge Wells was going to be harder than he had imagined.

If it had been India he might have stayed on, but not here. Unlike the politicians in Whitehall, Colonel Hutchins understood the threat posed by Si Pyo Lin's brother, by the Do Bama society and the Thakins. Though they were little more than student activists as yet, they had managed to forge irresistible links between independence, socialism and thuggery, and the Colonel didn't see how they could be broken. And although it was indeed idiotic of them to believe that the Japanese would be a better bet than the British – which was why the Governor dismissed them as idiots – it would not be stupid of the Japanese to use them as pawns.

He just hoped that Si Pyo Lin's firebrand of a brother would have the sense to make use of his sibling when the time came. For Si Pyo Lin understood that the key thing was to do the job. You kept order. You made sure there was enough coal for the railways and electricity for the sawmills, that ships were unloaded, oil exported and factories staffed. Your nationality and your politics were both irrelevant; it was getting things done that mattered. The young man hadn't had the education of some of his countrymen, a few of whom had even been to Oxford or Cambridge and joined the Indian civil service, but in the Colonel's opinion he was all the better for that. Still, it meant that instead of running the country, which he could be trusted to do and do well, he'd probably just end up as headman in his home village.

'Where's the village?' The Colonel asked. 'How far away?'

'Perhaps three hours, by car.'

The Colonel knew he meant in the dry season. When the rains came the roads would be impassable.

'Who runs the place?'

'There is an elder, but really it is the Saydaw, the head monk.'

'Capable?'

'Very capable, sir. It is a big monastery. Perhaps three hundred monks. Each Saydaw knows all of them well, so he chooses the most able of them to succeed him. It is his decision, but, you see, it is also the ancestors who choose, in a long line.'

The Colonel looked around. All this, the vast golden edifice, the towers and turrets and minarets which glinted in the evening sunlight, the marble floors, the bejewelled Buddhas, all this had been done by the ancestors of the monks who were sitting here now. Not so different from

the British army, he supposed; at least, ever since promotion
had depended not on wealth or birth but on merit. And just
as he sometimes felt the presence of all those who had gone
before him in the regiment, especially when he sat underneath
their portraits in his place, their place, at the head of the
table in the officers' mess, so here he sensed the generations
of monks who had built and preserved their holy of holies
over more than two thousand years. That was a thought, two
thousand years; it rather put the army in perspective.

He turned to Si Pyo Lin. 'Would you take me there? To
meet your parents and the Saydaw?'

★ ★ ★

They went in a Land Rover. Si Pyo Lin had said it would be
better than the Colonel's car, and indeed there were three
places where the road disappeared into fast-flowing streams
so Si Pyo Lin had to get out and walk on ahead, testing the
depth, one hand holding his longhi up and the other gesturing
to the driver to show him the best way through. At one point
he stepped into an unseen gully and went in up to his waist.

It was almost dark when they arrived, and as far as the
Colonel could see, the village was like ten thousand others:
houses made of woven palm leaves and surrounded by
bamboo enclosures where the oxen were corralled for the
night; white pagodas – the place was not rich enough for gold
– and three monastery buildings with, and this was the only
unusual thing, a football pitch and a pair of white painted,
regulation-size goalposts. He looked enquiringly at Si Pyo Lin
who grinned back at him. 'Yes, sir. It was me.'

The Colonel hadn't known. 'Are you any good?' he asked.

'Goalie, sir. I am a goalie. Some of the monks are very skilled and they practise shooting at me.'

The Colonel was amused. 'And do you have proper games?'

'Oh yes, sir. Highly competitive. There are ten teams in the district.'

'Which is yours?'

'Arsenal, sir. The Gunners.'

The Colonel burst out laughing. 'Not Manchester United?'

Si Pyo Lin looked shocked.

'Oh no. We don't like Manchester United, not in this village. We don't like the people from Hunaing, so they are the red devils.'

'Ah. It was you who named all the teams?'

'Yes, sir. And the pitches.'

'So this is Highbury?'

Si Pyo Lin was delighted. 'Yes, sir. Very fine pitch. Very good atmosphere because the buildings are close on three sides, fans at the windows. Old Trafford at Hunaing is out in the fields – no good at all.'

The Colonel realised that Si Pyo Lin must have organised all this and he was certain it would be well run. He made a mental note to donate a trophy, perhaps a replica of the F.A. Cup. It was entertaining to imagine a triumphant team lifting the Hutchins cup long after he was gone – gone in both senses of the word.

Si Pyo Lin's parents were a surprise. Although he couldn't have said why, the Colonel had thought they would be unassuming people, perhaps rather in awe of their important visitor. But there was no trace of deference as the father shook his hand and met his eye. And when the mother came out of the kitchen bearing plates of food she smiled at him with a light-hearted warmth, as if in memory of good times shared when they were young together. All in all, it was no surprise they had two such remarkable sons. Presumably the other son would not turn up, would not wish to greet the colonial oppressor – which was a shame, Colonel Hutchins thought, as what better way to get the measure of the man than to see him in his own home and with his own family.

Speaking in Burmese, the Colonel conveyed the high regard in which he held Si Pyo Lin and expressed appreciation for his dedication and skills. The father replied at some length until his wife stopped him with a hand on his arm and a shake of her head. Si Pyo Lin explained that his mother had realised the Colonel could not understand a single word of what was being said. The Colonel smiled at that, adding that his speech was a prepared one which he had learnt off by heart, finding it useful on many occasions. Si Pyo Lin translated, and they all laughed. Then he added that this time it was sincere, and with that he handed over his gift, an embroidery of the Shwedagon Pagoda most beautifully made with gold thread and river pearls.

'Embroidery is an ancient tradition in this country, I think,' the Colonel said.

'That is so,' replied the father. 'Though nowadays the art cannot compare with what was done in the days of the palace of Ava.'

'Indeed, much must have been lost with the end of the court of King Thibaw.'

'That is true. But you British are only the most recent of a long line of conquerors of this land, each taking the place of the previous rulers and each destroying what came before, as is the way of things.'

'I fear we have destroyed more than the vermillion gates and the red and gold umbrellas of the court. We have also taken some of the natural resources of the country.'

'As did all previous invaders,' Si Pyo Lin's mother added. 'But unlike them you paid for what you took.'

The Colonel smiled. It was both intelligent and generous to recognise that for all their faults the British had tried to behave with fundamental decency and honesty.

'No corruption.' She went on. 'I hope we will learn that from you.'

* * *

The monastery was immaculate: paths swept, woodwork painted, bells polished to an almost military shine. The Colonel raised his eyebrows. 'Three hundred monks,' said Si Pyo Lin, 'free labour'.

They were shown into the presence of the Saydaw who sat in a chair almost large and ornate enough to be called a throne. The man had presence, thought the Colonel. If he had simply been impassive and unmoving he might have been mistaken for a bully, and a rather stupid one at that, but his stillness came from some deep serenity and there was no doubting the intelligence in his eyes. Involuntarily the Colonel found himself bowing slightly and was surprised to receive a small bow in return. The two men met as equals.

Si Pyo Lin sat on the floor but a chair was brought for the Colonel. As he sat down he realised it was up to him to start the conversation; after all it was he who had asked for this meeting. But in the moment he felt uncertain, unable to find the words for what he really wanted to know. He rejected a number of possible openings as too conventional and too empty of meaning for this encounter, this man. Given permission by the Saydaw's serenity, he waited until he was moved to speak. When he did so, the words that came out of his mouth surprised him.

'What will it be like here, when we are gone?'

'Worse.'

It was not the answer the Colonel was expecting. 'Will you not run the area here, as well as the monastery?' he asked.

'I have power, but not that kind.' The Saydaw paused and opened the palms of his hands. 'The nearest hospital is fifty miles away – it might as well be in England. So one day I will build a hospital here: fifty beds, an operating theatre for eye surgery, a lab for blood tests, traditional medicine too. I can do that. But over the rice fields and the mines, the oil wells and the forests I have no power. And they will be destroyed by those fighting for them.'

'You cannot stop it?'

'Only an army can stop it. You are the army and you will leave. As I say, worse.'

The Colonel was moved. This monk, leading a life so different from his own, had grasped the value of the army and understood why he had felt that becoming a soldier was a noble calling.

The Saydaw went on. 'The flame of independence burns bright at the moment. That flame burns with the fuel of frustration, of idealism and longed-for pride. But what will feed it when you are gone? Greed and fear, the settling of petty scores, nepotism and revenge. Not good fuel. So the flame will die out. Then it will flare up again as a new invader arrives. Fire then ashes, fire then ashes, when what a country needs is a steady heat.'

Si Pyo Lin had sat at the feet of the Saydaw since he was a small boy but never before had he heard him speak in this way. And he knew it was the truth.

Then the Saydaw asked about the army – what was the essence of the training; how long was needed to create a disciplined force; what was required for the army to accept civilian authority? They were good questions and the Colonel realised how pertinent they were for the creation of a Burmese army after the British had left. At first the Colonel replied briefly but the Saydaw pressed him so in the end he spoke at length. When he had finished he felt it only polite to ask the Saydaw the same kind of questions. Si Pyo Lin expected to hear an outline of the Buddha's teachings but the Saydaw chose instead to tell the story of the Buddha's life. 'It is our inspiration, you see,' the Saydaw said at the end. 'An example to us all.' The Colonel took the point. It wasn't do as I say but do as I do. He liked that.

★ ★ ★

The Colonel stamped around his office in a fury. London didn't have a clue. They'd always treated Burma as a poor relation, as if the country had been taken in out of charity, placed at the foot of the table and then been pensioned off with a pittance. And now they were doing it again, sending out a new Governor who had never risen to the top, who hadn't been at Eton with Mountbatten and who wouldn't be able to get anything done in Whitehall however hard he tried. And he hadn't a clue about Burma. 'Read up the history on the boat over,' he'd said. As if that told him anything about the instability of the place at the moment, about the complex mixture of respect and loathing for the British, about the growing awareness that its Empire was crumbling and the Japanese were eyeing the spoils. And his books would tell him nothing about the people, their warmth and generosity, their quick cleverness and their profound respect for the monastic life. In fact, offhand, the Colonel couldn't think of a set of characteristics more different from those of the average Englishman nor less intelligible to someone who had spent his whole life in the British civil service. He lifted his eyes to the heavens at the thought of trying to brief the man.

And that was without even trying to explain something that was fundamental to every Burmese he had ever met. For all but a few, prostration before a statue of the Buddha was no empty gesture but a deeply felt reverence, and Buddhist teachings informed all aspects of their daily life. Every family had someone in holy orders and the ties between the monks and nuns and the lay people were a thousand times closer than in the West. It formed the bedrock of the whole society. And yet the new man would treat it all with a kind of polite indifference; the Colonel knew he would, for that is precisely how he himself had regarded it. Until he met the Saydaw, that is.

He had been impressed by the man, by his orderly running of the monastery, by his clear grasp of the political situation and also, the Colonel admitted it to himself, by a kind of holiness he had not encountered in vicars at home or army padres abroad. And in their conversation he had learned of the Buddha's renunciate path. He had never given such a thing any thought before, but if he had he would have dismissed it as idiotic. But now he appreciated that it might be necessary to give up everything in order to find a way to relieve the suffering of others; and there was undoubtedly something admirable about the Buddha's tenacity and steadiness of purpose. But what struck the Colonel more forcefully than any of this was the contrast between the evident power of his teachings – after all, countless millions were still following them two and a half thousand years later – and their patent implausibility.

On the journey back from the village he had plied Si Pyo Lin with questions. What could one possibly learn from paying close attention to the breath? In fact, how could the entirely passive practice of meditation achieve anything at all? And surely whatever monks and nuns might do in their monasteries could make no difference at all to the suffering of a mother who had lost her child or a young man gravely wounded in battle. The young man had a strong sense of the value of meditation and of the monastic life but his answers could not withstand the Colonel's relentless logic. 'I find I cannot explain,' he said finally, 'but am sure the Saydaw could enlighten you.' The Colonel thought that was a good idea and wrote him a letter with a long list of questions.

The reply came remarkably quickly and the letter was brief. Clearly the Saydaw had not found the questions difficult at all. The Colonel waited with some impatience for Si Pyo Lin to come to his office to translate. The young man read out loud. 'First, no one can tell you the answers to any of your questions – you have to do the practice to discover for yourself. Second, it would be ridiculous for you to do the practice – you are a Christian so you should follow Christ and not the Buddha.'

'Well, I'll be dammed,' said the Colonel.

Si Pyo Lin thought for a moment that he was about to witness one of the Colonel's rare, but terrifying, outbursts of anger. But instead he burst out laughing. 'Damn feller,' he said admiringly. 'Put me in my place, eh?' He strode round his office slapping at things with his baton then paused to look keenly at Si Pyo Lin.

'You do the practice, don't you – so you know the answers?'

'I suppose so, sir.'

'But you can't tell me. Because…because…' he was trying to find the words to express what he could only faintly grasp. 'Because it's not a belief, because a belief is something you have to take on trust. Because it's not logic either. It's a sort of…'

The Colonel felt trapped. He wanted an explanation but the only way to get it was by a route that was barred to him. And he hated being told he couldn't do something. As for being a Christian, it was true that he had attended church religiously all his life but he had never believed in God for one minute. So that didn't hold. In fact, none of it held. He didn't have to give in meekly. If he wanted to do the practice he was bloody well going to do the practice. And if that made him ridiculous, well, he didn't give a damn.

★ ★ ★

The Colonel's leaving party was to have been at the Pegu Club but as Burmese were not admitted he insisted the venue be changed to the Rangoon Gymkhana. An invitation arrived for Si Pyo Lin and his family. His parents thought they would go. It would be interesting to see inside somewhere they would never otherwise visit. Han Min couldn't believe they would even consider attending.

'You are going to pay tribute to your oppressor?'

'Not exactly,' said his mother. 'And anyway I'd have thought you'd be happy to celebrate his departure. It's what you want, isn't it?'

'Not his. All of them.'

'It's a start though, isn't it?' She never could resist teasing him.

'And if they are the enemy,' said his father, 'which I don't believe myself, then wouldn't it be a good idea to take the opportunity to get to know them better?'

'What?' Han Min almost shouted at his father. 'They came eight thousand miles to colonise the country without even a pretext of a justification and then they imprison people who dare to object. What more do I need to know?'

'Perhaps their merit,' said Si Pyo Lin.

His brother turned on him. 'You are so attached to them, to everything British, it's embarrassing. I don't know why you don't go back with the Colonel and live in England and wear a suit and smoke a pipe and go to church and drink tea all day with your beloved Huntley and Palmer's biscuits and have the pleasure of living with people who will always look down on you and consider you inferior and will make sure you never rise above being their servant...'

'While you will be so noble as to invite the Japanese to invade the country and despoil it. And then, when the British get rid of them for you, you won't even be grateful; you'll start complaining all over again, and when they finally leave for good, as we both know they will, sooner or later, you'll spend all your time arguing about communism and capitalism and how many seats in parliament should be allocated to different tribes so you'll hardly notice that the country is going to ruin through neglect, incompetence and disorder.'

'We'll be rich once we take for ourselves what the British took from us.'

'On the contrary. Wealth comes from stability and fair administration and you've no idea how to create either of them. You'll impoverish the country with your self-righteous speeches and self-indulgent theories.'

'Anyway you can't come to the party...' said his father.

'What do you mean I can't come?' demanded Han Min. 'I've been invited. I can come if I choose.'

'...because your friends might find out.'

He had a point, Han Min admitted to himself.

* * *

It all turned out much as the Saydaw had predicted. The Japanese invasion brought in a four-year rule of exceptional brutality, and Han Min and his colleagues were eventually forced to admit that it had been the most enormous mistake to side with them and think of them as liberators. The British and their allies, engaged in a desperate struggle against Hitler in Europe, still managed to muster the resources to defeat the Japanese, though with much loss of life, and shortly thereafter granted Burma full independence.

Han Min became a minister in the first government. All the senior positions in the civil service went to a small elite, men from wealthy families who had been sent to England for their education, so the best he could do for his brother was to get him appointed as the manager of the Irawaddy Shipping Company.

Before the war this had been an enormous enterprise running over six hundred ships, all built on the Clyde, dismantled, transported, and re-assembled at the shipyards in Rangoon. It was also vastly profitable as it formed the main means of moving people and cargo through a country which had less than a thousand miles of single-track railway and roads which were impassible for much of the year. The river, on the other hand, ran the whole length of the country and plumb through the middle at that, bringing oil, teak and minerals down to the docks and manufactured goods up to Mandalay and beyond. More important still, between the branches of its vast delta lay the most productive rice fields in the world. Over three million tons a year were exported, and all of them on the boats of the Irawaddy Shipping Company.

But when Si Pyo Lin turned up on his first day at the famous headquarters on the Strand, he found a ghost of the organisation it had once been. Six of the fourteen panelled rooms had gaping holes in the walls where the building had been hit by artillery fire, and the cabinets with all the company records, the best part of a hundred years of paperwork, had gone up in smoke. Rumour had it that the British had scuttled all the ships to prevent them falling into the hands of the Japanese and no one seemed to know how many of them, if any, had been refloated. The Superintendent of Transport, a political appointment with absolutely no experience of shipping or administration, gave a rousing speech to the staff, told Si Pyo Lin that he had every faith in his ability to get the company back on its feet, and departed in his chauffeur-driven car. The four clerks, all new to the job, looked to him for instruction. He could think of none that made any sense, so he told them to go home and come back the next day.

He sat down in despair. He had been waiting for this moment since he had first joined the Colonel's service all those years ago, waiting for the day when the responsibility for the administration of some key sector of his country would be in his own hands and for the opportunity to become an exemplar to those he would train to be good administrators. He had imagined himself in neat offices which would be run according to orderly procedures, where the staff knew their precise roles in the organisation and attended to their work with diligence and proud impartiality. He had supposed he would work closely with his political master who would be equally devoted to Burma and its people, helping it to modernise and become prosperous again. Instead he found himself in a bombed-out room with no money, no budgets, no records or accounts, no ships and no idea how to create a functioning enterprise from scratch. Nothing in his training had taught him how to do that.

So he sat at his desk long into the night, planning his escape. The country was in chaos. He could change his name, go to some remote part in the north and get a job as a schoolteacher; no one would ever know. They'd assume he'd been killed, somewhere somehow, like so many others in the past ten years.

It was nearly dawn before he got up and walked out of the office, not knowing where he was going. He found himself climbing the deserted steps up to the Schwedagon Pagoda. That brought back memories of the Colonel and the sight of him taking off his socks and stuffing them off into his pockets. The Colonel had not asked questions, nor had he complained or stood on his dignity, but without a moment's hesitation he had done what was right. And then Si Pyo Lin knew that he could not run away.

He climbed to the top and sat before the Buddha which had been his particular favourite since he was a boy. Slowly he composed himself and asked for help.

★ ★ ★

The next few months passed in feverish activity. Some of it was planned. He spent his evenings going round all the dockyards of Rangoon in search of ships and every weekend being ferried to any small creek where one might be moored or beached. He found six which had escaped being scuttled and survived the fighting with the Japanese and which needed only minor repair and restoration. Through a network of friends and relations, and friends and relations of theirs – for there was no local administration any more – he found out where there usable landing stages, and started to draw up the basic routes and timetables of his new service. Some of his progress was the result of happy accidents, as when more than eighty uniforms of the captains and pilots were found in a disused warehouse. And some came about as news of his activities spread and experienced pilots, crewmen and shipwrights turned up looking for work.

He knew that he couldn't do a tenth, a hundredth, of what had to be done so he decided to put all his resources into getting one route up and running first; then his masters would see what was being done and he would be able to ask for the money and support the shipping line really needed. So it was only four months after that despairing night in the office that the first scheduled trip on the first recovered ship set off from Rangoon to Bagan carrying rice, oil and machine parts. Bunting fluttered in the breeze, a brass band played (not everyone approved of the colonial overtones) and the Superintendent made a speech. It was front page news the next day, Han Min was congratulated by his fellow ministers and one of the most senior civil servants, an Anglo-Burman who had elected to stay and help the nascent nation, invited him for drinks in the Strand Hotel.

When Si Pyo Lin walked somewhat nervously through those famous door and looked around him, wondering how to find his host, the concierge came up to him immediately and escorted him to a small room off the bar. A tall thin man in a grey flannel suit, starched collar and silk tie rose from his chair and held out his hand to be shaken. 'Si Pyo Lin? Delighted, delighted. Hearty congratulations, young man. You've done well, very well. Sit down, do. Drink? Whisky, beer?' Si Pyo Lin chose a beer – he hadn't had one since before the war. It was cold with a slight head, clear underneath, absolutely delicious. It felt like an initiation.

'Imported, I'm afraid,' said his host. 'We will get our own brewery up and running, definitely. Not a priority, though.

Not like your shipping line. Speed is of the essence there. Security. There are threats to the government, you see, insurrections, rebellions, communists. Might have to move troops and supplies in your ships. And in any case, we need them in order to rebuild the economy. Don't have to tell you how important that is. Food and essential supplies where they are needed; exports in order to earn currency. None of that can happen without shipping. The Irawaddy! The great river. The artery of the nation. So your ships are the blood, the lifeblood of our country.'

Si Pyo Lin felt dizzy. The luxurious surroundings, the impeccable clothes, the studied eloquence, the unexpected praise, the sense that he was being drawn into a confidence and made part of the bigger picture, all of it was intoxicating and it went to his head. So when his host spoke briefly again and then stopped, clearly waiting for a response, Si Pyo Lin had no idea what was being asked of him. 'I am sorry,' he said. 'Would you mind repeating your question?'

With a smile came the response, 'I am not surprised. It isn't easy to hear something completely unexpected. What I asked was – what do you need?'

Si Pyo Lin's mouth opened and shut but no words came out.

'I know. The answer is everything. I'm not asking for detail. But how long would it take to get all six ships working?'

Si Pyo Lin considered. It was no good taking on staff if he didn't have time to train them. No good commissioning ships without crew, or fuel, or places where they could unload cargo. No good making a promise he couldn't keep. He shook his head. 'I am sorry, sir, but I could not do it in less than six months. And then I would need...'

'Good man, good man. Excellent. And whatever you need, just come to me.' He held out a business card with two addresses and three phone numbers. Si Pyo Lin couldn't imagine how you could have three phones. 'Let's not get the Superintendent involved, eh? Heart's in the right place, I'm sure, but he's a politician. No idea how to get things done, have they? Just you and me; that'll get things moving. Alright?'

'Alright,' said Si Pyo Lin, thinking how inadequate that word sounded.

And his host was as good as his word. First, Si Pyo Lin was given a budget and it was bigger than he had dared hope. Then he was given the power to sign chits on the government. And finally, when the new state-owned oil company said they could not supply enough fuel for six ships, Si Pyo Lin rang one of the numbers on the card, and it was delivered within a week. Many years later, telling the story of those early days, he couldn't help smiling at his naivety.

Looking back on it, he could only feel sympathy for that enthusiastic and dedicated young man. He could see how easy it was to overlook the first signs of the troubles that were to engulf him. After all, he had managed to get the ships fully operational in under six months, he had been singled out for special treatment, and in any case he was working so hard that he had no time to reflect on the occasional hiccup.

And indeed the first one seemed trivial enough and it was a pure fluke that he even found out about it. He had news one day that his mother had fallen ill and might not survive long. Tears filled his eyes. He was too busy to leave his work but he could not bear the thought of her dying before he had seen her one more time. He realised he was just in time to catch the next ship to Bagan, and he would have a couple of hours with her before catching the next one back. He had to go.

The crew did not know him and the captain was too busy to notice that their employer had come on board. Nor, as evening fell, did anyone see him looking surreptitiously under the tarpaulin on the aft deck. There should not have been a tarpaulin there, nor any cargo underneath it, and especially not any cargo which Si Pyo Lin was not expecting. There must have been more than a hundred bicycles and not one of them was on the bill of lading. He waited until the ship returned to Rangoon and met it on the dockside. There again, on the deck, was an unauthorised cargo.

The captain met Si Pyo Lin's eye. 'For my uncle,' he said. 'It does no harm. And perhaps you and I could come to some understanding?'

Si Pyo Lin was outraged and sacked the man on the spot. The other captains came to him and asked him to reconsider. 'Are you all carrying illicit cargo?' he demanded, and saw from their eyes that they were. 'It is theft from the company, theft from the government and therefore theft from the people. Anyone carrying such cargo in future will not only be sacked but will be charged as a criminal.'

Han Min telephoned him. 'I think you're getting a bit too big for your boots, little brother,' he said.

'Are you asking me to condone corruption?'

'I would not call it corruption. Everyone helps their family, it is natural. I helped you to get the job if you remember.'

'I can't let the line be run for personal profit.'

'I am not saying it should be, but remember how we do things. Take an older brother's advice. Sometimes it is better to be flexible.'

A few months later Si Pyo Lin received a request to alter the sailing times of a ship from Mandalay to Rangoon in order to accommodate a large wedding party.

'Why can you not catch the ship at the scheduled time?' he asked.

'The festivities will not finish until too late.'

'Then change the time of the festivities. I cannot run a shipping line to accommodate the needs of every passenger. No one would know what time a ship was leaving or arriving. Impossible.'

So it was a bit of a shock to receive a telephone call later that day from the Superintendent ordering him to change the schedule. Si Pyo Lin argued, but to no avail. So he telephoned the first of the three numbers on his card, spoke to the man's secretary and was put through.

'Ah, Si Pyo Lin, yes, yes, I have heard about this little brouhaha...'

Si Pyo Lin was shocked that the matter had reached ears so high.

'...and I quite understand your position, naturally. Must be an awful nuisance changing things ad hoc like this. And I suppose you think that if everyone started doing it...'

'Exactly, sir.'

'Quite. But still, there is always a time to bend the rules a little and I rather think this is one of them. VIP and all that.'

'But, sir...'

'I think you have your answer,' he said, and put the phone down.

The last thing that tripped him up was, to Si Pyo Lin's mind, the most galling. It all started when one of the ships had been hit by a coaster which swung out of control as it left the dock. Under pressure, a joint between two plates under the ship's waterline had cracked, and the captain decided that the leak was too severe to allow him to sail. Passengers and cargo were disembarked and the stricken vessel towed to the shipyard.

Si Pyo Lin spent a frantic day getting passengers and perishable cargo re-booked on another ship which was detoured to pick them up, and then arranging new schedules based on the shipyard's assurance that the repairs would take no more than two days at the most. But on the third day he arrived at work to the news that the ship not still not been repaired or launched, and that his new and carefully constructed schedule was in tatters. He exploded. For the first time in his life he took a taxi.

When he arrived at the shipyard he marched into the manager's office.

'I do not ask for an explanation,' he almost shouted at the man, 'nor an excuse. The work must be done and I will not leave until I have seen it done.'

The manager was a fat man who didn't even attempt to lift himself from his chair as he said, 'Impossible.'

'Why impossible? Not impossible. Two days maximum, I was told. The schedules are arranged. I demand the work is done. If you won't do your job I will find someone who will.'

'No matter who you employ you will get the same answer. Impossible.'

Si Pyo Lin almost danced with fury. 'Two days work...'

'Oh, the work is done. It is the launching that is not possible.'

'What?'

'It is not astrologically propitious.'

'What! I don't care if it is propitious or not. You think I can run a shipping line in accordance with the orbit of heavenly bodies! This is the twentieth century. Do it.'

'As for myself, I might – though I would not like to answer for the consequences. But that is not the point. The men won't do it.'

Si Pyo Lin was not to be denied. 'Take me to them.'

He stood on a stepladder and addressed the workers. He started by appealing to modernity and to the part they were playing in creating a new Burma, but they were unmoved. So he tried pleading, speaking of the disruption to the service all along the Irrawaddy, about the people who were missing family events and the factories which were running out of supplies. It made no difference. Finally he blustered, saying that they could be sacked if they did not carry out orders. At that the twenty-three shipwrights, with no more than a glance between them, turned as one man and walked out.

The manager looked at him. 'What do you propose now?'

Si Pyo Lin walked back to the office composing the speech he would make on the phone to his superior. It ranged widely, speaking not just of his present difficulty but of the demands of a modern state; it poured scorn on superstition and spoke of the discipline of a chain of command. By the time he arrived it was perfect. He called the number on the card and poured it out.

'Yes, I see. Of course. Leave it with me.'

Si Pyo Lin put the phone down, rejoicing in his righteous indignation. While he waited to see the swift executive action he so admired, he got on with re-writing the terms and conditions of carriage. But the expected phone call was not from his superior but from the Superintendant. With no preamble he simply told Si Pyo Lin that as from that evening he would no longer be employed by the Irrawaddy Shipping Company and that a new manager would take his place with immediate effect.

For the next three days Si Pyo Lin rang the number on his card, but the secretary regretted that his call could not be put through. He rang Han Min. 'I cannot help you, little brother,' he said. 'And you can't say I didn't warn you.'

Si Pyo Lin went back home, to the comfort of his parents and the village where he grew up. He told his father the whole story and the old man listened patiently, nodding every now and then to show he understood, but saying nothing. Si Pyo Lin expected praise but he got none. Perhaps the old man simply could not grasp the demands and pressures of running such an important organisation and could not see the full merit of his actions. Maybe he could think of no advice which would be appropriate to a man who had held high office.

After three days the Saydaw summoned him.

'What are you going to do now?' he demanded.

'I don't know.'

'What is your father's opinion?'

'I don't know.'

'Have you asked him?'

'No.'

The Saydaw looked severe. 'Your father is the first person you must ask. It is respectful. In any case he is a man of insight and experience and he knows you better than anyone.'

So after the family meal that evening Si Pyo Lin sought his father's advice. The old man sat in thought for some time and then started. 'Your great-grandfather was at the court of Ava, you know. He was a scholar, a pyinnya-shi, educated at the Bagaya monastery at Amarapura, and he advised on court ceremony and precedence.' Si Pyo Lin shifted in his seat. The faded photograph of his ancestor in full court regalia hung in pride of place in the main room; this was a story he had heard many times before.

'Note,' said his father, 'that patience is not your strength. This is relevant.' He paused to see if Si Pyo Lin was paying full attention. 'And at the court there was constant danger.

Everyone's job, everyone's life indeed, depended on the whim of the king. There were always people who were jealous of those who held office or were offended at decisions they had made. They dripped poison about them into the ears of the king, hoping he would replace them with members of their own families. To survive, as your great-grandfather did, demanded a complex set of skills and understandings and it required a honed instinct. As a sailor can sense the slightest shift in the wind, so a courtier senses the slightest change in favour or disfavour.

'You think it is not like that now; that we have learned to do things differently; that the British taught us how to organise and manage in this modern world. I don't deny their skills and understandings but they are not ours. Your Burmese superior is not like your Colonel; he is more like your great-grandfather. Any senior courtier would have sensed danger in your decisions and would have taken action to protect himself. Your great-grandfather himself would have dismissed you in order to protect his own position. If you want to do more than work in the fields for the rest of your life you will have to learn the old ways.'

Si Pyo Lin felt rebellious. That all died with the court of Ava, he thought, overwhelmed by the power of the British. Surely it was better to learn their ways as he had learnt from the Colonel.

His father saw the resistance in his son. 'Soft bamboo,' he said. 'Soft bamboo. The British have no bamboo in their country so they do not know this.'

For the next few weeks Si Pyo Lin studied his country's history and the way it had been run through a network of minor nobility who had personal allegiance to Thibaw himself, and who administered justice, collected taxes and presided over the innumerable festivals and ceremonies that linked the ordinary people to their rulers. All that had been swept away. When the British invaded the country without a shred of legitimacy and deposed Thibaw, forcing him into exile, they destroyed a complex system of government and imposed one that was utterly alien to the country and its culture. That was the one, Si Pyo Lin realised, that he had been at such pains to copy. Now the British were gone, was it any surprise that the last thing his countrymen wanted was to be ordered about by a Burmese man who was aping their conquerors?

Si Pyo Lin went to the Saydaw and offered to do the administration needed to build the hospital he had always wanted. 'The old way,' he said with a smile. By the time the Saydaw died it was already the largest hospital in the region, though not yet as big or as well equipped as he had planned. When Si Pyo Lin retired from his post as head of the hospital, many years later, it had over a hundred beds, employed more than twenty doctors of both Western and Traditional Burmese medicine, and had the best-equipped operating theatre outside of the capital.

As for the Colonel, in retirement he practised his meditation with the relentless consistency with which he did everything. To his considerable surprise it led him to Christianity. For in the silence of his daily practice he came to realise the truths the Saydaw had said he would discover for himself, and that those truths were no more and no less than the teachings of Christ. He died peacefully in the sure and certain knowledge of eternal life in the kingdom to come.

11

Gall Bladder

When to quit

AT THE END OF THE BOARD MEETING THE Chairman asked the new Managing Director to stay behind for a moment. The boy looked so young, still in his early thirties, that Henry couldn't help wondering if he was up to the job. Still, Charlie was able, no doubt about that. His previous company had been on its knees when he'd taken it on and he'd turned it round and made it hugely profitable. They weren't in that much trouble, nothing like, but Henry knew they were stuck in their ways and losing ground on their competitors. They needed something new and Charlie was the only one they'd interviewed who had offered anything more than cliches and platitudes. He'd been eloquent about the need for a more co-operative culture in the organisation and he'd talked the panel into believing it. Henry wasn't entirely convinced.

'You won't have to worry about the Board,' said Henry. 'They won't care what you do as long as the figures look good. And it won't matter much if the middle managers don't get it, at least at first. But the Department Heads – frankly you're asking them to change their spots. They won't like it and they might fight; or they might simply make sure they undermine whatever you do.'

'I thought of showing them what happens when they don't consider collaboration,' Charlie replied. 'The real costs. It's an exercise devised by Anatole Rappaport, I met him once. Brilliant man – though, ridiculous as it seems, the only thing I can remember from the whole conversation is that he pointed out that the buttons on the sleeve of my suit were a remnant, I think that's the technical term, in the same way as the coccyx is a remnant of a tail we once had.' Charlie held up his arm. 'Look. They don't even unbutton.'

Henry smiled. But if that was the kind of thing Charlie was going to use to win over the Department Heads, well, he'd get eaten alive.

* * *

Charlie stood in front of the oriel window. 'Let's start with a simple game,' he said. Because the light was coming from behind him they couldn't quite see the expression on his face so they weren't entirely sure how to respond. Roger wanted to say, 'Oh goody, a game – well worth taking a whole day off work and coming to a bloody country house hotel for.' Elaine crossed her legs and tucked one foot behind the opposite ankle as she always did when she got ready to defend herself. Lesley and Keith exchanged meaningful glances for this was a confirmation of what they had suspected when the meeting was announced: 'Oh God, that means paintball,' he had said.

'Or kayaking,' she added.

'Teams. Bonding.' He grimaced, thinking of the waste of time it would be and how he'd have to take work home at the weekend, again, to make up for it.

'Sharing,' she said with a shudder.

The others did their best to look enthusiastic. It was early days and most of them still wanted to make a good impression.

'I hope you'll enjoy it,' Charlie continued. A few of them smiled at him to show their willingness to enjoy themselves if that was what the new M.D. wanted. 'And the game will introduce what I hope will be the key theme of the day and of our work together in future.'

'I have here,' Charlie waved a small folder, 'two first-class air tickets to Pisa and a voucher for a week at the Hotel Splendido in Portofino, probably the most elegant hotel in Europe. Clarke Gable used to stay there and Greta Garbo, Graham Greene and Nancy Astor, the Duke of Windsor and Wallis Simpson. The clientele these days isn't quite up to that standard, but then again if it was, they wouldn't let any of you through the door.' A few titters at this. 'I'm putting this package up for auction. As usual, the highest bidder will get it, but there is a twist. Whoever is the underbidder, that is whoever makes the penultimate bid, will have to pay too, and pay whatever he or she bid.'

Roger groaned inwardly at the 'he or she'. He couldn't bear political correctness.

Charlie paused briefly.

Henry, who was sitting on an upright chair at the back of the room, looked at Charlie with a mixture of admiration and apprehension, much as he had looked at his daughter at the start of her first run-up to the vaulting horse. It would be spectacular if it worked and the most dreadful crash if it didn't.

'Is that clear?' Charlie continued, looking round the room. 'Any questions?' No one spoke. 'OK. Now, what am I bid?'

A silence fell. They were all trying to work out what was expected of them. Sally raised her hand. 'A thousand pounds,' she said, in a clear confident voice. She hadn't worked out a strategy; she simply wanted to be seen as a good sport, one willing to join in and get the ball rolling.

'It's worth far more than that, Sal,' said Keith.

'It's an auction, Keith,' she replied. 'You're supposed to try to get it as cheaply as possible.'

'Still,' Keith wanted to show he'd done the sums, 'I reckon you should have started at four thousand, or a bit below.'

'Thanks for the advice.'

'It's not advice really. I'm just trying to play the game the way it's...um...isn't it?' He looked to Charlie, who gave no sign that he had heard this appeal to his authority. 'I mean, we don't want to be sort of taking advantage, not really doing it properly, if you see what I mean, because I don't think...'

'Oh, for God's sake, five thousand.' That was Roger. He didn't particularly want the holiday. He couldn't quite see his wife Yvonne in such a place, not with her voluminous patterned dresses and a tendency to go bright red in the sun and peel, but he'd spend the money gladly to stop Keith flopping about like a wet fish.

'Six,' said Nick who was starting to enjoy himself. He saw what Roger was doing and saw too the opportunity to hurt him a bit. Here was a chance to make him into the underbidder, so Roger would have to pay five thousand pounds for the luxury of saving Keith from himself; which was well worth six thousand pounds to Nick any day of the week, and especially on a sunny day in a posh hotel conference room.

'Seven,' Roger almost shouted. He was damned if he was going to let Nick get away with it again, looking down on him all the time, treating him like an idiot.

A silence. Their personal animosity filled the room like the stench from a drain.

'Why don't you go together, you two?' said Jennifer sweetly. 'After all, you're both going to have to pay now.'

Marcus, sitting in the deep armchair by the side of the fireplace, put his head back and laughed out loud. For a moment Roger looked offended, then he too started to laugh. He'd judged it pretty well, Jennifer thought; the rueful laugh of a good sport. Elaine uncrossed her legs, ready to get up.

'Ten. Ten thousand.' That was Nick again. As far as he was concerned, the logic hadn't changed. Whatever he bid, Roger would still be the underbidder and he'd end up out of pocket for nothing. That was the point.

Roger turned red. Another silence. The tension was starting to get to them all. Lesley was biting her lip, Henry noticed, and Marcus had got up from his chair and was standing, hands deep in his jacket pockets, straining at its hand-stitched seams.

'Fifteen.' Roger glared round the room. 'I can afford it.'

A few of them looked down, not meeting his eyes. This wasn't good.

'But...' Keith shook his head and waved his hands in a gesture of despair. 'You know, Roj, it really isn't worth that much. I worked it out and it doesn't come to...'

'It is to me. It's worth it to me.' Roger spoke through his teeth.

Another silence.

Jennifer cleared her throat. She looked at Charlie and in a sweetly reasonable voice said, 'Aren't you going to do that going, going, gone thing?'

'Alright,' he replied. 'Going, go…'

'Sixteen.' The voice came from the back of the room. For a moment they weren't quite sure who had spoken, then they realised it was Lesley.

'Are you out of your senses, woman? Don't you see what you've done?' Roger always blustered when he was angry.

'Oh, I don't think it was Lesley who did it,' said Jennifer.

Marcus let out another of his booming laughs.

'Why? I mean, why?' asked Keith of no one in particular.

'Well, if you're asking me,' said Lesley, 'I just didn't want it to end quite yet. I'm enjoying it, as requested, and I think we need a bit longer to get to the theme of the day, as our M.D. put it.'

If this was intended to draw a response from Charlie, it failed. Henry noticed how still he was, not reacting, not betraying by word or gesture what he wanted from them.

'Tell you what, Roger,' said Elaine, 'if you bid again, I'll go halves with you.'

But Roger was long past the stage when he could recognise a lifeline when it was thrown to him. 'No, thanks,' he said.

'Your funeral, Roger,' she replied.

'Oh, I don't think so.' This was said with real hostility.

'She was only trying to help,' said Keith. 'I do think you might…'.

'What the hell's it to do with you?' Roger shouted.

Silence. No one was supposed to show anger even if they felt it.

'If I might bring us back to the matter in hand.' That was John, the finance officer. They all looked at him, wondering what on earth he could have to say. 'The auction is still in progress, I think? Then I bid twenty thousand.'

They couldn't believe it. For one thing John very rarely spoke in meetings except to explain the accounts, and for another they weren't aware that he had any issues with any of them which might explain this recklessness. He sat in his own office, in his own world, and did his own thing, taking no part in office politics. So what was he up to? They'd always thought him dull but sound. They'd have bet their houses on it, and now, they realised, they'd have lost them.

None of them was under any illusions any more; they were in unknown territory and they didn't have a clue how to find their way home.

'You sure, John?' Elaine asked gently.

He nodded.

It seemed to break the spell. Somehow, the game had come to an end, though in a most unexpected way. It was as if, rather than picking up the ball, John had plucked the goalposts out of the ground and wandered off with them over his shoulder.

Lesley, however, had been paying attention. She was well aware that John's bid had left her as the underbidder at sixteen thousand. 'Twenty-five,' she said.

'You're crazy.' Keith stood up in his agitation. 'Just do the bloody maths, woman.'

'Actually I did,' she replied. 'You think women can't do sums, don't you? This bid makes me a thousand better off. Work it out.' She paused. 'I'll wait.'

'She's right,' said Jennifer. 'She's in for sixteen thousand anyway, so for an extra nine – that's the twenty-five she's bid – she gets a holiday worth about ten.'

'That's true as far as it goes,' said Elaine, leaning back into the corner of the sofa, 'but it doesn't go far enough. All I have to do is outbid her and it won't work.'

They all turned to her.

'Don't look at me! I'm not daft enough to spend in excess of twenty-five thousand pounds for a week's holiday in a poncy hotel, especially when it would cost me less than half of that to book the damn thing myself.' She picked her bag up from the floor and put it on her lap. 'I can't imagine what our new Managing Director must be thinking of us all, but I don't suppose he's over-impressed with our financial acumen – though I'm impressed by his. At the moment he's standing to make a profit of about thirty-five thousand pounds for an investment of ten thousand and about fifteen minutes' work.

'And at the very least,' she went on, 'it settles one question conclusively. Possibly, some of us came here wondering if our new M.D. had what it takes. No, let's be frank, none of us thought he had a hope in hell. We assumed he'd be full of well-meaning but absurdly uncommercial schemes, that he'd want us all to have hug-ins and go round honouring each other and he'd ask us to come to meetings with some object from home which means a lot to us so we could share our feelings about it, and we'd have to grin and bear it and fawn in public and sabotage it all when his back was turned, which we would have done very…'

'I say, Elaine, I don't think that's quite fair…'

'Oh, shut up, Keith.' She banged her fist on the arm of the sofa. 'Quite fair? You've just lost the match six–love and you're complaining about a bad call from the line judge.'

Marcus laughed again.

Elaine swung round to face him. 'And I suppose you think you got away with it by standing aloof there at the side and not committing yourself and smirking at how idiotic we've all been, but you don't win anything by refusing to play, and you don't make any difference by being superior and smug and smarmy in your fancy suit which cost far more than any man should spend on his clothes.'

John, who was sitting next to her on the sofa, patted her on the back and said, 'Bravo.'

'I wonder, Mr Chairman,' asked Jennifer, 'if there is a limit to this thing? I really would like a coffee.'

'Going, going...'

'Thirty,' said Elaine.

The silence which followed this went on for well over a minute. It was broken by Frank. 'There's your answer,' he said. 'Don't you see? It'll end when we stop bidding. Is it possible,' he looked round the room, 'in the name of all that's holy, that we could agree to stop? Come on. Hands up if you agree to make no more bids. Roger? Keith? Jennifer? Thank you. Marcus? Lesley? Oh, come on, Lesley, for God's sake.'

'You forget, Frank, that at the moment I'm the underbidder,' she said. 'You're asking me to spend twenty-five thousand pounds for nothing.'

'Well, I'm in for thirty,' said Elaine.

'We'll just have to pool it then,' said Frank. 'There's nine of us, and the cost of both bids together is fifty-five thousand. That's just over six thousand each which, frankly, is cheap if it gets us out of the hole we've dug for ourselves.'

One by one, they agreed.

'All done then?'

'Except for one thing,' said Sally. 'Who gets the holiday?'

'That's obvious.' Jennifer was heading for the door. 'There's only one winner. The auctioneer, right? If we decide he gets the holiday, which would be the only sensible decision we'd have made all morning, he'll get fifty-five thousand pounds from us for nothing.' She paused by the door. 'Come on. Can anyone seriously disagree that he's the winner?'

No one spoke.

'Going, going, gone,' said Charlie.

12

Liver

The Navigator

I T WASN'T COLD, SITTING ON THE BOW OF THE outrigger as dusk fell over the Pacific, but he wrapped himself in a blanket all the same. He needed to be contained, isolated from the others, inward.

They had been sailing for twenty-six days and nights and every day he'd altered course half a dozen times, but the course he was going to set tonight would be the vital one for they were approaching the crown of the ocean, the centre from which its currents radiated in every direction, so it was here that a mistake of a mile would throw them irretrievably off course, missing their island by who would ever know how far or in which direction.

He could feel them all sitting in the main hull looking at him with respect, even awe. They all knew that he'd never been to sea, never been to the island, but none of them doubted he would lead them there for they knew his reputation; and perhaps they were also half aware that if they lost faith in him they might as well jump off the boat and have done with it.

With his left hand he held onto the smooth wood of the prow and with his right he grasped the thick tight rope stretching to the masthead. He felt proud of them all. They'd done well on that beach beneath the redwoods, building this craft. It had sailed well, lasted well, was fit for its purpose. Now, was he? He'd never doubted it before. That's why most of the tribe called him arrogant.

As a child he would chase a deer far from the campground, not to catch it, just for the pleasure of knowing its ways, when it twisted to turn downhill, where it hesitated and paused to look back at him, how it jumped the brushwood. When he was a little older he'd lashed three logs together and rode them down the great river through canyons and rapids no one else had dared traverse. As a young man he'd walked for days in one direction to see what lay there, reaching snow-covered mountains in the east and gazing over the sea in the west, sights which none of his tribe had ever seen. And he'd always found his way back. He didn't think it was arrogant to claim he could, to know his own skills; besides, what they didn't understand is how hard he'd worked to hone them.

It had started with a sense of smell. The camp sat on earth which had a distinctive odour, and he discovered that a strip of that earth ran for about ten miles north-west; he only had to pick up the scent and he could follow it home without fail. The smell of the bushes told him how high he was and whether or not there was water close under the surface. Animal droppings warned of dangers; he could smell if there was fear in them.

Then he started to develop his other senses. Soon, from the cloud formations above, he could tell the lie of the land twenty or thirty miles away; only one particular structure could generate those shapes and no others. He could tell the course of unseen valleys by feeling the twists in the wind that funnelled out of them. And he'd learned to trust his sixth sense, a kind of awareness that came when he'd gathered information from all his other senses and held it together, at the same time, until every piece fitted, made a pattern, made sense. And he could only do that, he'd discovered, when he was calm and still inside. Hence the blanket.

The first star, when it came out, should be just a fraction to the left of the masthead. He looked up and there it was, in exactly the right place.

The six senses weren't enough on their own; there was something else he needed. He only discovered it when the tribe moved to a new campground while he was away scouting. He'd never been to the new place but he knew the area and didn't think he'd have any difficulty finding it. A few days later, when he'd finished scouting and wanted to go there, he discovered he had no idea how to find it. Without a mental picture of where he wanted to go, as a kind of magnet, he had no inner compass and was lost. It felt terrible.

He never told anyone that he'd cheated. He had to go back to the old campground and follow their trail from there, like any half-asleep brave. He was ashamed of himself. But he was also wise enough to know that it was a lesson worth learning; thanks to that, he'd asked the old woman for the clearest possible description of the island before they left. He saw it now, in his mind's eye, ahead of him, tugging, the pull of it a faint pressure through his body and into the hull. He'd respond to it, but not yet, not quite yet.

The gentle breeze held steady and the boat glided along, heeling minutely, barely disturbing the water beneath him. He leaned forward and dipped his hand into the sea, held it there for a few moments, then lifted it out and tasted the salt water on his fingertips. He was preparing, the way an athlete warms up or a cook lays out ingredients; getting himself into the swing, becoming familiar with things so that there would be no fumbling, in the moment, under pressure. The darkness deepened and a softness in it told him of cloud, thick cloud, to come. He'd hoped for moonlight, expected moonlight. Tonight of all nights he needed to see the ripples of a current shining silver, the contrasting blackness of an eddy, the oily slick of a deeper flow – he needed all that to make the right decision at the right time, and he was going to be denied it. Was it so much to ask? Had he ever sought help? Why was it always so hard for him? Why?

He'd always felt excluded by the tribe. As a child he'd sensed the jealousy and resentment which was directed at him, and it had pushed him out and onto his journeys. It had got much worse since he had started to warn them of the threat. On his travels east he'd seen how another tribe was flooding westwards towards them. Even the best of them cut down the forests – the forests! – while the worst of them... well, the brutality was unimaginable. The chiefs of his own tribe hadn't understood. 'Maybe they'll stop before they get here,' they'd said, 'and anyway, we're sure they'll be friendly, like us. Why not? There's plenty for all.' Some thought that by his warnings he was claiming to see the future, the prerogative of only a few rare beings and he certainly wasn't one of those; others believed he was simply bidding for power – 'frighten people enough and they will follow you'. Nearly all of them thought he held himself aloof and regarded himself as superior, and they disliked him for that. It had hurt but he'd kept the pain well hidden; getting angry with the chiefs would have been disrespectful; getting angry with the others was beneath him.

Only one person understood, a woman who had been old when the elders were babies. She summoned him to her presence one day and from under the hides on her litter a skeletal hand had emerged and grasped his. She told him that the chieftains were idiots because they took no interest in the legends and myths of the tribe, their stories: in fact they'd forgotten them. Yet without the guidance they contained how were they to navigate the dangers that lay ahead? 'If we choose leaders like these we deserve to die out,' she told him without a trace of bitterness. Then she recounted everything that had been handed down, the accumulated wisdom of a people. It took her ten days and the last legend was for the darkest of times; for now.

A sharp clatter broke the silence. With a wave of fury he knew who'd disturbed him – that clumsy, ugly, stupid woman knocking something over again; it was always her, waddling around like a stork with a stomach ache, eating twice as much of their precious rations as everyone else. Damn her. How could he be expected to gather all his powers of concentration if she couldn't even sit still?

He knew he shouldn't move but he couldn't resist it. He swung round as if to glare at them. They wouldn't be able to see his face in the dusk but he knew they'd be watching him and the change in his shape would be as shocking to them as a scream. He wanted to frighten them, to hurt them; he wanted them to cower at his rage and to beg and plead with him inwardly – they wouldn't dare approach him – not to abandon them even though they knew they deserved to be abandoned.

As his fury flowed out of him like lava, he saw it was limitless, that its source was as deep and as wide as the very centre of the earth, and that there was an inexhaustible supply inside him which would sear and scar anyone who happened to puncture the thin skin which held it in. And it was justified, every drop of it, because of all the pain and hurt and betrayal he'd suffered and all the strain of carrying this bunch of wastrels and incompetents – well, who else would follow him but the gullible and the stupid, the feckless and the greedy? – carting them over the hills and guiding them over the ocean to a paradise they weren't worthy of, none of them. That they were literally the seed of a great tribe – to be planted, watered, cultivated, to blossom and bear fruit – was laughable. No wonder he'd always been alone, travelled alone; he couldn't have done it, any of it, if he'd had to carry this hapless weight on his back.

He gave a start, as violent as if he'd been woken from a deep sleep by icy water on his skin. He had no idea, none at all, how long he'd been in this reverie of rage, discerning nothing in the darkness around him. Perhaps they'd passed the place where he needed to alter course, or it might be right here, at exactly this moment; he wouldn't know. All he could see, hear, smell, taste, touch or comprehend was his anger.

He wouldn't regain his senses without letting go of the fury and the ill-will, that was clear; and he needed those senses to find the island. But was he willing to let them go? He didn't know. They were precious to him, certainly. Then he started to laugh at the absurdity of it all. There was no real choice at all. Even if he'd wanted to, he couldn't imagine how to let go of his rage.

He felt stirrings in the other hull. First his fury, now this manic laughter. They were bemused, nervous. One of the children started to cry and the noise was shut off so suddenly it must have been by a hand clamped over the child's mouth. Poor child, afraid, miserable, wanting to be back with the sweet smell of earth and leafmould, with the comfort of knowing where his home and his bed were. It wasn't so different for him: he too was bereft and he could almost feel a hand stopping him crying. In fact, it wasn't so different for any of them; they'd all been frightened, bullied, belittled; they'd all felt the pain of being separate, unloved; they all longed for safety and comfort. He'd done it to them as it had been done to him – that woman, so terrified of his anger that she dropped things all the time; he'd made her suffer as he'd been made to suffer. That child was crying for all of them. 'Let the child cry,' he said to himself, and he cried.

As he wept he knew it wasn't personal, that it wasn't his grief he was feeling but everyone's. And so he saw that the same was true of his rage: he didn't need to claim it, to pull it to him as a greedy man will seize a delicacy, didn't have to desire it or possess it like a lover, nor did he have to believe that it belonged to him as a recompense for all the hurt. Like the grief, it was everyone's. For the first time in his twenty-nine years he saw that he was simply a part of life, one of its unknowably vast variety of manifestations, like a tree or a crab, a beetle or a bullrush, even a wave. Life had taken the form of him, temporarily, as it took the form of everything else temporarily. And feeling that he was no different, that he would die as everything else dies, his senses returned, and they were more acute than ever before.

He wiped his eyes, looked round, sniffed the breeze, touched the water and called over to the man at the helm, his voice as light and unconcerned as he felt. 'About ten minutes or so. Watch for a time when the current pulls strongly to the right, then ceases – that'll be the zenith of the ocean. Helm hard over then, pull the sail well in, take her left as fast as you can to carry us through the current on the other side. I'll call again when we're there, but you'll feel it.'

He heard people relaxing in the other hull, moving stiff limbs, making beds, getting food. After the change of course he crossed over the connecting beam and joined them. About half an hour later the clouds parted and the moon shone out, but he barely glanced around because he knew where he was, and once you know there's no need to check.

After that he was never known by his birth name, but out of respect was always called The Navigator. The tradition held, and even today the official title of the President of the island is The Navigator, and the story of how he came to have that title has not been entirely forgotten.

Appendix

The organs in Chinese Medicine

THE NOTION THAT AN ORGAN HAS A SPIRIT IS entirely alien to Western medicine and may seem peculiar to readers who are not practitioners. The word spirit is not a terribly good translation precisely because there is really no equivalent in English to the Chinese term; it certainly has nothing to do with religion or even spirituality. The nearest is something like a quality of being. Think of the differences between a tiger and a koala bear, both mammals, or a robin and an eagle, both birds; and between people of course, some of whom seem overwhelming while others appear to shrink into a smaller space than their bodies occupy. So it isn't hard to imagine that each of the organs has its own quality, that the heart and the stomach, for example, are different not just because of differences in shape and tissue, but because of what you might call their intrinsic and unique natures.

1. Lungs

When a baby is born the organs of the body will have been working for months – all except the lungs. That first breath, as the child goes from a world of fluid to a world of air, activates the lungs and inaugurates a system of energy throughout the body. When all is well, the energy that fills the lungs flows from them round the body, organ by organ, until it reaches the liver. After that it then flows back up to the lungs, completing the cycle which will power the human being for the rest of his or her life. On the other hand, when all is not well and for some reason there is a delay in energy reaching the liver, then the organ won't be able to cope with the new demands put upon it and the baby goes the typical yellow of jaundice.

During this flow round the body each organ has a period of two hours when it receives a boost of energy, and for the lungs it is from 3.00 to 5.00am. Accordingly, monks and nuns in every spiritual tradition I know wake for their first prayers or meditation at 3 o'clock – they want to catch their lungs at their best. On the other hand, if you want to be asleep at 3 o'clock but often wake up, as many people do, it is a sign that the flow from the liver back up to the lungs isn't getting through as is should; hence, like pain or any other major disturbance, it wakes you up.

The word 'inspiration' is a clue as to why this is so. It implies that there is a very close connection between breathing in, on the one hand, and suddenly knowing exactly what to do or say, suddenly appreciating a reality hidden behind the daily busyness of life, on the other. In the Eastern traditions it is an awareness of life as it really is, seen in a moment; in the Western religious traditions it is an awareness of God. So the function of the lungs in Chinese medicine is not merely the mechanical task of bringing oxygen into the body and expelling carbon dioxide; it is to keep us closely in touch with what inspires us and what is precious in our lives. Those who are depressed or in grief, who have lost this, tend not to breathe properly.

And finally there is a close connection between the lungs and the large intestine. It seems an odd partnership, one taking in the purest and most unmaterial of substances and the other expelling smelly waste, but there is a good anatomical reason for it. The diaphragm is a thick band of muscle which cuts the body cavity in half horizontally – above are the lungs (and heart) and not far below is the large intestine. The main way we breathe in is by pushing the diaphragm down (which pulls air into the lungs just like sucking on a straw). And as it goes down, rhythmically, it massages the large intestine, and that helps to move the stool along. So it is not surprising that those who breathe very shallowly often suffer from constipation; the colon is not getting a helping hand from the lungs.

This is a good example of something that you will encounter throughout these brief sketches of the organs in Chinese medicine. Thousands of years of clinical observation has produced a view of the body which, although very different from our modern Western view, accounts for what is often seen in normal life.

2. Large Intestine

The organs in Chinese medicine are seen more as a set of functions rather than as distinct pieces of tissue. So while in both systems the large intestine is concerned with creating and expelling faeces, the Chinese give it a wider role and significance. For just as the organ gets rid of dead cells and the remains of food which no longer contain any nourishment, so it should allow us to let go of anything which doesn't sustain us any more – which may be a relationship, a job or even a belief. In all these instances, holding on for too long is seen as a kind of constipation; it not only preserves what will gradually become toxic but it also means there won't be room for anything new. Hence, in the old texts, the large intestine is often described as being responsible for change. It's a nice idea; that only by being willing to let go can we really take in.

And there is another aspect of the work of the large intestine to which the Chinese give wider significance. As the faeces pass through it, the large intestine absorbs fluid and vitamins back into the body. These vitamins, mainly K, B12, thiamin and riboflavin, are found in tiny amounts but they are essential to health, and historically we could not rely on getting more of them regularly. Hence the notion that a key function of the large intestine is to find what is special and precious. Its job is like that of a gold miner who has to separate out tiny grains and nuggets of something immensely valuable from enormous amounts of rock. And finding gold metaphorically is also about finding a speck of something which is worth far more to you than all the rest. So someone who finds herself suddenly unable to respond to a much-loved piece of music or to a favourite view, who no longer feels her spirit lift at the things that have always meant a lot to her, may be seen as suffering from a malfunction of the large intestine.

Knowing what really matters is the other side of the coin of knowing what not to keep, and the large intestine at its best can do both.

3. Stomach

In pre-scientific Western thought the behaviour of the natural world was seen as arising from the interplay of the fundamental elements – earth, air, fire and water. The Chinese had much the same idea (though they added an extra element) and when they applied it to medicine it meant that each of the organs was believed to have something of the quality of one of the elements. The nature of the earth element is obvious from common expressions such as mother earth and earth mother – it is all about care and support, about sustenance and nourishment. As the main function of the stomach is to break down the food we eat and turn it into a substance which can be absorbed into the body, it is naturally linked with the earth element. Think home and hearth, a full store cupboard, a flourishing garden and Sunday lunch with all the family around the table.

Mothers are acutely aware of the needs of their children so it is natural that one of the key characteristics of the energy of the stomach is to be aware of the needs of others. The ability to acknowledge and understand another's distress, to sympathise with his or her predicament, comes, in this system of medicine, from a well-functioning stomach. It is an example of the Chinese way of seeing the organs as having functions which are not only physical but mental, emotional and even spiritual too.

This can be clearly seen in the names of some of the acupuncture points on the body which are directly associated with the stomach. One of most powerful of these is called 'People Welcome', which to me conjures up the image of friends coming into our kitchen after school for my mother's warm compassion almost as much as for her home-made cakes. And in case this makes the stomach seem a little mundane, another point, an inch or so on either side of the umbilicus, is called 'Heavenly Pivot'. There are many ways to interpret this evocative phrase but I think it is a reminder that the stomach is at the centre of everything; imagine an enormous see-saw with heaven at one end and solid earth at the other – the stomach is the point exactly between them which holds them in perfect balance.

Perhaps this is the real essence of the stomach. It knows all about soil and rain, milk and flour, grazed knees and hurt pride, but at the same time it can have an awareness of that which – though it has different names in different cultures such as God or the Dao – is another kind of reality.

4. Spleen

There is something mysterious about the spleen. Most people have a rough idea of the shape and location of the other organs – heart, kidneys, lungs – but only those with medical training can do the same for the spleen. In Western medicine its functions are hard to pin down too, having to do with cleaning blood and producing blood cells on occasion. In Chinese medicine it is also seen as having an important role in the creation of blood but it has far wider functions (though admittedly they encompass the work of the pancreas, which sits on top of the spleen, as well).

The main function of the spleen is transformation. This involves taking things in one state and changing them into another. There is often something magical about this, like combining flour, water and yeast, adding heat, and producing bread. Similarly, it is astonishing that whatever we eat, foods as different as fish and chips, apples, broccoli, rice or cheese, can all be transformed every day into things as different as blood, hormones, bones and hair.

As ever, all this applies to the mind as well as the body, so the whole business of transforming an idea into an action is the work of the spleen. At its best it gets organisations built and staffed or supplies delivered to inaccessible disaster zones; but if it is weak, then a lot of worrying happens but nothing much gets done. Being stuck in a rut is a typical failure of the spleen.

And there is another level to this too. Going back to the example of bread, notice that the combination is extremely unlikely. Going to the immense labour of grinding up corn until it is no more than a powder, then mixing it with water to make a paste to which you add mould – it is almost unimaginable. And there you see the power of the spleen at its very best, for it provides the power to perceive hidden potential inherent in a situation and makes it possible to envisage what would normally be regarded as utterly implausible.

Finally, many of the examples I have used are to do with food. That is because, as with its close neighbour the stomach, the spleen is linked to the earth element and that in turn is the source of most of what we eat. More widely, it is the earth which holds everything in place. This may seem to contradict the idea of transformation, but it all depends which time scale you have in mind. Every day we trust that the earth will be completely stable and not move under us – earthquakes are devastating – but in geological time, of course, the earth has moved massively, lifting mountains thousands of feet into the sky.

5. Heart

There is a curious discrepancy in the Western view of the heart. On the one hand it is always associated with love, and especially romantic love, while on the other it is regarded merely as a pump. The Chinese view is more coherent. It sees the heart more simply as the organ which rules over all others.

The idea of ruling derives from an analogy between the body and a nation state. In old texts the heart is often called the Emperor, and in ancient China the Emperor was vital to the well-being of the state. It wasn't that he had overt power, nor that he took any part in the management of affairs, but he had a crucial ceremonial role. If he performed the prescribed rituals in the traditional way and at exactly the right time, then all would be well. His doing so would provide the reassurance of order, stability and predictability, and that then allowed all the other organs of government to do their work properly.

It isn't so far-fetched to see the heart in this way. For one thing the regular rhythmic sound of the heartbeat penetrates every cell of the body and without it the other organs don't function well – arrhythmia often leaves people feeling weak, breathless and distressed, and it can have serious consequences. And then there is the regular supply of blood from the heart which carries the oxygen and nutrients on which all the organs depend.

Rituals and their regularity used to be an important part of everyday life, mainly because so much depended on the changes of the natural world. When to plant crops, when to harvest, when to regard a child as adult, when to fish for trout or catch a tide at its zenith – these were all key moments, and rituals showed you what to do when. Hence the idea that it is the heart and its regularity that makes sure that the right things are done at the right time and the right words are said on the right occasions.

It would be a mistake to think of this as a matter of useful but dull routine. On the contrary, being in harmony with what nature demands and allows, celebrating the flow of life as it changes, and knowing an appropriate response to it all, is what brings joy to the mind, a sense of ease in the body and a sparkle to the eyes. This sparkle is the unmistakable sign of a heart which is working well and which is open and available to others. Perhaps it is this joy and this ability to connect and communicate from the heart that we in the West are really speaking of when we talk of love.

6. Small Intestine

The small intestine is a tube, but what a tube! It is about twelve feet long on average, occupies a good deal of the middle and lower abdomen, and it has a remarkable talent. Semi-fluid and partly digested food comes into it from the stomach, which is just above. The food then passes down the small intestine which absorbs nutrients into the blood stream through its wall. That's how nourishment is taken into the body to energise and sustain it. Anything that is not nutritious or is positively harmful is passed on down to the large intestine to be expelled. In other words, the small intestine's great talent is to be able to distinguish what, in all that mushed-up food, is good for you and what is not, and then to separate the two of them out from each other. Endless choices – absorb or reject; nourish or protect? – and all of them important.

If it doesn't work properly – for example, by rejecting what is good for you – then you are bound to be thin, tired and vulnerable to illness; young women may lose their periods and be unable to conceive. If it accepts what is in fact bad for you, then the consequences range from what is often called an upset tummy to serious and potentially lethal food poisoning. And if the small intestine loses confidence in its ability, throws up its hands in despair and decides that the safest thing to do is simply to reject everything – that's diarrhoea, which can also be serious if it goes on too long.

So the key issue is one of judgment, and in particular judgment about what to absorb into the body and, of course, the mind too. Watching distressing images on the news or seeing violence on film or television raises the question – can the small intestine cope with deciding, frame by frame, what to absorb? And is the long-term effect of bombarding it with such images to weaken it, so it becomes progressively less able to nourish and protect? And then there is the level of emotions. It is perfectly reasonable, in Chinese medicine, to think that the small intestine of a woman who always seems to fall in love with men who treat her badly must be unwell. The same may be true of people who insist on refusing help from others.

Modern life is certainly a strain on the small intestine. Faced with an enormous range of products such as toothpastes of different sizes, prices and chemical compositions, the small intestine may find the choice bewildering. Then there are the chemicals and additives in much of our food, and it simply hasn't had enough evolutionary time to recognise them and their effects. And flicking through apps on a smartphone or tablet constantly engages it in at least an effort to know which one to use. And if it is weakened by all this, perhaps it will be less able to make good decisions about what will sustain us – and future generations.

7. Bladder

In our culture we tend to see the world as things. So we talk about a fist as if it were an object when in fact it is a movement (after all, where does your fist go when you open your hand?); and we say 'it is raining' when there is really no 'it' at all, just raining happening. So the Western view of the bladder is of an object, about the size of an avocado pear, which simply fills with urine, holds it and then discharges it. The traditional Chinese view is very different.

In that view there always the sense of flow, of movement and change; perhaps the oldest book in the world, and certainly one of the most influential, is the Chinese Book of Changes. Accordingly, the organs are seen not just as a physical part of the body but also as responsible for the organisation of flows and functions. The body has an enormous amount of fluid in it (apart from blood) and it has to flow in an orderly way; otherwise, for example, the eyes will not be lubricated, there will be no saliva to help break down and pre-digest food, and there will be no sweat to help the body cool down. It is the function of the bladder to make sure that enough fluid, and not too much, gets to where it has to be.

So the channel which carries the energy of the bladder is not confined to the lower abdomen – on the contrary, it is by far the longest in the body. It starts in both corners of the eyes by the nose, then runs in parallel lines up over the head, down the back quite near the spine, then down the back again a bit further out, before finally running all along the legs to end on the outside of the little toe, by the nail. In short it reaches every part of the body, as it has to if it is going to manage the accurate distribution of fluids throughout.

As I have mentioned before, each organ is associated both with an emotion and also with one of the elements.

The element for the bladder, obviously, is Water; less obvious is that the emotion is fear. But imagine the terror you would feel if you had been on the coast of Aceh or Sri Lanka when the tsunami struck and devastated everything in its path. Too much water. But running out of water is terrifying too; you know you can survive a long time without food but not without water.

And finally there is the spirit of the bladder. It makes sure that what has to be done is done, whatever difficulties or obstacles stand in the way. But it is more than a kind of dogged persistence; there is in it a sense of rightness, of making sure all that everything is being managed properly for the benefit of the whole.

8. Kidneys

The moment an egg is fertilised it divides. What was one becomes two, and from then on there are the contrasting qualities of life, what the Chinese call Yin and Yang – light and dark, wet and dry, heat and cold, male and female. In this world of duality one kidney is regarded as Yin and the other Yang, and between them, in the middle of the spine, is an acupuncture point called Gate of Life. The idea is that as soon as there is a connection between Yin and Yang then all the myriad forms of life can be generated. Hence, for the human being, the kidneys are seen as the source of our inherited constitutional strength, and are fundamental to our growth and development.

There is a compelling wisdom about this. It sees the way we develop as a bit like the way a tomato seed grows only into a tomato plant and an acorn grows only into an oak. So the kidneys provide the sense of a person's particular destiny and the power and energy to realise it in a lifetime.

This might manifest in a number of ways. One is through sheer willpower. Some years ago, for example, a climber fell thousands of feet and sustained terrible injuries. He could not be rescued but somehow, over the course of five days, managed to crawl his way out of a crevasse and back to safety. As he told of his ordeal (in an unforgettable film called *Touching the Void*) his body was still and his face almost expressionless; he betrayed no fear but only an implacable will. That implacable will comes from the kidneys.

The power of the kidneys might manifest instead through an instinctive and unconscious recognition of the purpose and meaning of a person's life; a kind of co-operation with the inevitable. Reading the biographies of great reformers like Florence Nightingale and Elizabeth Fry, it seems that they had no choice but to do something which was highly unusual for women of their time and class. And when a reporter asked Mahatma Ghandi, 'What is your message?' he received the reply, 'My life is my message.' That's the authentic voice of the kidneys.

The climber forced himself to endure and survive by a conscious act of will. The will of the reformers on the other hand, though it also enabled them to persist and endure, had a softer quality to it, one of accepting one's fate with all its consequences. There are two contrasting aspects to kidneys but together they always relate to something deep within us.

9. Pericardium

The heart is so important that it needs to be protected. The rib cage gives the outer layer of protection and forms a barrier to all but the knives of skilled assassins – the thrust has to be upwards at just the right angle. Then the heart is surrounded by a fluid-filled sack, called the pericardium in Western medicine, which insulates it from physical shocks and from anything harmful which may be wandering about the chest cavity. And finally, in Chinese medicine there is a third and entirely different layer of protection, confusingly also called the pericardium. It's a bit like a venetian blind which opens and shuts in response to the intensity of light coming from outside – except that you can't see it or touch it. That's because it has an energetic not a physical presence.

We're quite used to such things – when we are about to get to an automatic door we cross an unseen barrier of energy which triggers its opening, and contactless cards trigger payment in essentially the same way. The ancient Chinese thought that we guard our hearts with something of the sort – opening the heart's protection in the presence of those who love us and closing it when there is a threat. We all know what this is like. I could practically feel my heart open to my daughters when they were babies, and I certainly know the sensation of closing my heart when I am with people I find uncongenial, aggravating or even downright threatening. The first is accompanied by feelings of warmth, affection and communication, the second by a cold, hard quality, as if I am insulating myself from the other and making sure that nothing he or she says will have the power to hurt me.

And the existence of a pericardium that is not working well does account for two common experiences which can be very damaging to health. One is leaving the heart open at a time of danger or threat – what we call heartbreak causes more than emotional pain, though that is bad enough. It weakens the power of the heart and that has a consequent effect on all the other organs; hence heartbreak is often a precursor to illness and the onset of disease.

The opposite, keeping the heart closed when what is being offered is love and support, is not so obviously damaging but it stops the heart being nourished, and stops the heart providing emotional nourishment to another. The end result is a person who is starved of the human contact we all need. It is no way to live and in the long term the result is also illness and disease.

Most of the time most of us can open and close our hearts appropriately but we can lose the capacity to do so. How can the tyrant start to act toward his enemies with common humanity? And how can someone who has been badly hurt emotionally learn to open up to new love? It isn't easy to do it without some help, and one form this can take is by treatment of the pericardium through acupuncture points with such evocative names as Inner Frontier Gate and Palace of Weariness.

10. Three Heater

Whereas there are organs such as the stomach and the liver in both Western and Chinese medicine, even if they mean rather different things in the two systems, there is no Western equivalent of the three heater. That is because it is a not a specific body part but a set of functions. To us it seems odd, therefore, to call it an organ, but the Chinese always see the organs primarily in the light of the activities which have to be carried out in the body, so it causes them no difficulty.

And it is quite clear that the functions of the three heater are essential. All the other organs only work well within a pretty narrow range of temperature around 98.4°F, and that temperature has to be held steady day and night and in wildly different climates. So the primary task of the three heater is to register when the body is being threatened by heat or cold and then to activate a selection of an enormous range of mechanisms – sweating is the most obvious example – in order to bring body temperature back to within acceptable bounds. You can think of it like a thermostat in a house which switches the boiler on and off as it senses deviations from the set temperature.

And the reason it is called the three heater is that there are traditionally three body cavities – the upper chest above the diaphragm, the middle abdomen between the bottom of the rib cage and the umbilicus, and the lower abdomen below that. And if the three heater is working well, then all three cavities will be more or less the same temperature. So if, for example, the lower cavity is cold, then you would expect problems with urination, perhaps painful periods and so on.

As this organ is concerned with keeping a steady temperature it is naturally associated with the fire element. And this explains why it has a huge part to play in regulating body fluids. If, because the three heater isn't working well, the body overheats, then fluids will evaporate; the mouth and eyes will go dry, joints will start to creak for lack of lubrication and so on. Similarly, if there is not enough heat in the body, then fluids will start to accumulate and congeal; limbs will swell, toxins won't be expelled and there may be seemingly endless phlegm in the nose and chest.

In short, the three heater provides a stable, warm environment which allows everything else to work well. So typical signs of a three heater which needs some support are those people who are constantly falling in and out of love, or who start new hobbies or projects all the time but do not persist with any of them, or those who are elated one day and low the next – manic depression is a severe failure of the three heater. More generally, the three heater helps a person to recognise and respond to his or her own boundaries, whatever they may be. We call it 'knowing one's limits' and it is the wisdom of the three heater.

11. Gall Bladder

The gall bladder is a very small organ tucked in right next to the very much larger liver, and its limited function of storing and releasing bile into the digestive system is rather overshadowed by the numerous and essential activities of its neighbour.

Both are associated with the element called wood, which is to say the energy of all vegetation, including trees. And the most striking thing about this energy is that it pushes unstoppably upwards. Over time, tiny shoots grow into tall trees, weeds will break through concrete and plants impeded by a fence or barrier will deviate crookedly round it and keep going. Taking this as a metaphor for human life, the Chinese see the liver and gall bladder as providing the forceful, driven energy that gets things done.

They regard the ability to get things done as having two distinct aspects. First there needs to be some vision or plan, which is the work of the liver, and then there has to be the detailed decision-making that implements the plan, which is the province of the gall bladder. These activities can be done either with flexibility or rigidity – another metaphor taken from wood – and in relation to the gall bladder's decision-making that reveals a kind of power on the one hand, and a kind of pathology on the other.

First the power. Given our limited knowledge of the complexity of life, and the fact that things change all the time, many decisions which seemed good when they were made turn out to need revision. The ability to be flexible, to be willing and able to adapt and find a better course of action in the light of new circumstances is a great strength. It means that the plan can be realised in spite of difficulties, even if by a very different route than was first envisaged. It takes courage to have the kind of persistence which adapts, adjusts, accepts setbacks and disappointments and carries on all the same; to say someone has a big gall bladder means, to the Chinese, that he or she is brave.

Now the pathology. Insisting on implementing the plan as first conceived, refusing to alter decisions made even when they are patently not helping, affects people in different ways. Some will end up with a frustrated fury that circumstances have changed or that others have failed to understand the plan or have stopped it working. This kind of rage over-stimulates the whole body and leads to long-term consequences for health – chronically high blood pressure, for example – as well as alienating friends and colleagues. Others, when things go wrong, choose to see the whole plan as flawed and impossible, so they become apathetic and give up. Both of these responses show that the true and healthy energy of the gall bladder has become weakened or distorted.

12. Liver

In Western thought, all ideas come from the brain which is in the head. Not so in Chinese medicine, which attributes different kinds of thoughts to the work of different organs – concentration comes from the spleen, memory sits in the heart, decision-making is a function of the gall bladder and so on. The liver's particular ability is to plan. And planning requires a vision of what will happen or what will exist in the future; it is thinking strategically and taking the longer view.

Hence the notion that the liver is involved with vision in all senses of the word. While we are busy with everyday tasks it is the liver which keeps an eye on our higher aims in life and tries to ensure that we don't lose sight of them.

As you can tell from what I have written so far, it is practically impossible to talk about the liver without speaking of eyes and sight; indeed, the channel which carries the energy of the liver upwards passes right through the centre of the eyes – hence a number of eye complaints are regarded as dysfunctions of the liver, and the colour of the whites of the eyes reveals a liver damaged by alcohol.

What the Chinese call the spirit of the liver also has a long-term quality to it, for it lasts beyond the death of the body. It is a bit like what we would call a person's fame or reputation. For most people, it survives perhaps two of three generations – grandchildren and great-grandchildren may remember them and what they have done. But for exceptional men and women like Mozart or Florence Nightingale, their liver spirit is so powerful that it lasts for centuries.

All this needs a powerful energy to fuel it, and there is none stronger than that of the liver. It has the unstoppable force of a rambler rose climbing ever higher or a seedling breaking through the surface of the soil. This energy has an upward and outward movement and it sometimes comes out as a shouting voice and a waving fist, and then we call it anger. As an emotion, we tend to associate anger only with rage and violence but it has a very benign side too. It can come out as a refusal to accept injustice and unfairness, said with a quiet but firm 'no'. It can come out as an appropriate and unshakable self-esteem. And it can come out as the necessary force to impel badly needed change.

Much of this is summed up by the name of an acupuncture point. There is a twenty-four-hour flow of energy round the body, starting with the first point on the channel which carries the energy of the lung and ending with the last point on the channel which carries the energy of the liver; and then the whole cycle starts again. That last liver point looks ahead to the start of something fresh and is the pre-cursor to new life. It is called Gate of Hope.

References

Introduction: Spirit

Kaptchuk, T.J. (2000) *The Web that Has No Weaver*. Chicago, IL: Contemporary Books.

4. Spleen: Transformations

For the fossils in Canada see Gould, S.J. (2000) *Wonderful Life: Burgess Shale and the Nature of History*. London: Vintage.

5. Heart: Mr Spencer

The history of the bicycle is beautifully told in Penn, R. (2011) *It's All About the Bike*. London: Penguin.

6. Small Intestine: Lady Mary

The fullest modern biography of Lady Mary Wortley Montagu is Grundy, I. (2001) *Lady Mary Wortley Montagu: Comet of the Enlightenment*. Oxford: Oxford University Press. There are various editions of her letters. I mostly used O'Quinn, D. and Heffernan, T. (eds) (2012) *The Turkish Embassy Letters: Lady Mary Wortley Montagu*. Ontario: Broadview Press.

Keats, J. (1817) Letter to Benjamin Bailey (22 November).

7. Bladder: The line

The story of the line and its parcels draws heavily on Bailey, R. (2009) *Love and War in the Pyrenees*. London: Phoenix, and on Nichol, J. and Rennell, T. (2008) *Home Run*. London: Penguin.

8. Kidneys: Twins

The misplaced hermit crab and the oysters who were doing their best are brilliantly described in Kingsolver, B. (1997) *High Tide in Tucson*. London: Faber and Faber.

9. Pericardium: Opening the gate

There is a Meeting House at Colthouse in Cumbria which looks much like the one in the story, and Satterthwaites have lived in the area for hundreds of years. The rest is fiction.

10. Three Heater: Soft bamboo

For the Irawaddy Shipping Company see Laird, D. (1961) *Paddy Henderson: The Story of P. Henderson & Company*. Singapore: Outram.

11. Gall Bladder: When to quit

An inspiring book on the subject of Game Theory is Axelrod, R. (1990) *The Evolution of Co-operation*. London: Penguin.

Appendix: The organs in Chinese Medicine

For more information on the functions of the organs in Chinese Medicine, see Kaptchuk, T.J. (2000) The Web that Has No Weaver, Chicago, IL: Contemporary Books, and Hicks, A., Hicks, J. and Mole, P. (2004) Five Element Constitutional Acupuncture. Edinburgh: Churchill Livingstone.